DIABETIC DELIGHTS

Festive recipes the entire family can enjoy!

CONSULTING EDITOR: GINGER MUSCALLI, R.D.
CHIEF DIETITIAN, THE JOHNS HOPKINS HOSPITAL

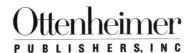
Ottenheimer
PUBLISHERS, INC

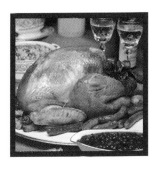

INTRODUCTION 4

FESTIVE ENTREES 7

SCRUMPTIOUS SIDE DISHES 29

TASTY TRIMMINGS 51

HOLIDAY DESSERTS 57

CELEBRATION PUNCHES AND
BEVERAGES 81

INDEX 87

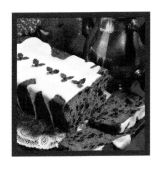

INTRODUCTION

When we designed this cookbook, it was primarily to offer those with diabetes a vast selection of delicious holiday meals. In fact, the recipes in this cookbook will delight *everyone's* taste buds—whether diabetic or not. The recipes on the following pages for tasty appetizers, scrumptious main courses, and tempting desserts combine the special requirements of the diabetic menu with taste-tempting recipes that will delight every dinner guest.

People with diabetes, with the help of their doctors and registered dietitians, will have already established their meal plans, based upon their individual dietary requirements. While some diabetic meal plans can tolerate small amounts of sugar or alcohol, others cannot. All the recipes in *Diabetic Delights* include food exchanges to make meal planning easy. You may, of course, further adapt these recipes to your particular plan by using some of the menu and cooking tips that suit your needs.

Now, holiday meals can feature delectable dishes everyone can enjoy!

Ginger Muscalli, RD LD
Chief Dietitian,
The Johns Hopkins Hospital

YOUR MEAL PLAN

The following step-by step suggestions will help you follow your meal plan as closely as possible.

1. Plan each day's meals at one time. This will help you keep track of your prescribed exchanges.

2. Always use measuring utensils or scales to guarantee accurate portion sizes.

3. Always start with the main entree. Then if necessary, increase or decrease the portions depending on the number of exchanges you are allowed. For example, if a recipe says 1 serving equals 3 meat exchanges, and you are allowed only 2 ounces of meat or 2 medium-fat meat exchanges, you should decrease the portion size to 2 ounces.

4. Calculate the exchanges from the starch/bread list. Again, adjust the portion size to fit your exchange if necessary.

5. Continue selecting recipes/foods that can be used in your meal plan from the remaining vegetable, fruit, milk, and fat exchange lists.

PORTIONS & FOOD EXCHANGES

If the serving size recommended is too large for your planned exchanges, you can divide the serving and the calculations to yield the correct portion. For example, a $^1/_2$ cup serving of Apricot Stuffing equals 2 Starch/Bread exchanges. You are allowed 1 Starch/Bread exchange, so your serving size would be $^1/_4$ cup.

If you would like a larger portion, multiply the calculations.

For greater ease in planning your meals, check off your exchanges when you select your recipes.

COOKING TIPS

ARTIFICIAL SWEETENERS

Artificial sweeteners are an option for diabetics. Remember—there are differences among the various artificial sweeteners. Be sure to read the label to determine the sugar equivalent. The amount to use may vary from brand to brand.

ASPARTAME (NutraSweet®) can be used to sweeten foods and beverages that do not require heating. Aspartame decreases in sweetness when exposed to heat, and it does not provide the bulk and structure for baking that sugar does. One teaspoon of NutraSweet® is as sweet as approximately 8 teaspoons of sugar.

SACCHARIN can be used in recipes even if heated. It should be added at the end of the cooking process because it tends to turn bitter if exposed to a high temperature. The sweetening power of saccharin depends on the brand used.

Low-calorie or non-calorie sweeteners should be used in moderation. If you have questions about a specific artificial sweetener, contact the manufacturer.

FAT

While all food categories should be included in exchange groups or a meal plan, remember that fats are high in calories and should be measured accurately. Here's a "baker's dozen" tips to decrease the number of fat exchanges in recipes:

1. When preparing a recipe, try using less fat than the recipe recommends. NOTE: This may not be appropriate for some baked goods.

2. Select lean, well-trimmed cuts of meat. For example, 85% or higher lean ground beef, and meats graded "select" have less fat than "choice" or "prime."

3. Trim all visible fat from meat and poultry prior to cooking.

4. Remove the skin from all poultry. Although poultry can be cooked with the skin to retain flavor and moisture, it should not be eaten.

5. Drain the fat when cooking ground meat.

6. Cook meats on a rack to allow fat to drip away. Be sure the rack has a tray under it to catch the fat.

7. Avoid frying foods and consider cooking methods that do not add fat. For example, bake, roast, broil, steam, grill, or microwave.

8. Season foods with herbs, spices, and "butter flavored" sprinkles instead of oil, butter, or margarine.

9. Use a non-stick cooking spray to brown, stir fry, or to grease the cooking dishes.

10. Serve gravies, cream sauces, and butter sauces on the side for adequate portion size control.

11. Choose low-fat dairy products such as skim milk, 1% milk, nonfat powdered milk; low-fat cheeses such as mozzarella and cottage cheese, and plain, low-fat or nonfat yogurt or light sour cream.

12. Use two egg whites in place of one whole egg for cooking.

13. Read the labels of nonfat or low-fat products to determine the actual calories per serving.

It may take awhile to find the right balance when changing fat ingredients in recipes. Allow for experimentation time to suit your individual taste requirements.

Planning in advance can make your holiday more enjoyable. Keep the following points in mind when you approach special-occasion cooking:

● Assemble, measure, and prepare all ingredients before starting to cook. This will save you preparation time once the recipe is ready to be mixed.

● Add special touches to your meals. Garnishing is an easy way to add color and make a meal attractive. Add parsley, radishes, and carrot curls to entrees or vegetable dishes. Strawberries, grapes, and orange slices can be used as garnishes for desserts or fruit dishes. Frozen fruit in ice cubes or ice rings can spruce up beverages or punches.

● Go easy on meat garnishes. Several recipes throughout this cookbook call for sausage or bacon. Although these are high-fat meats, they have been calculated into exchanges. Remember to drain bacon well on layers of paper towels.

Sausage can be boiled in water and browned without additional fat.

● Be sure to have containers with tight-fitting lids on hand if you plan to freeze leftovers. Never freeze food while it is still warm. Label the container with the date, contents, and serving portion. Remember to check the dates when you are ready to use the food and arrange containers to follow the rule "First In, First Out."

FESTIVE ENTREES

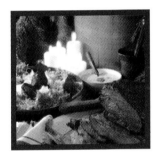

A golden goose or turkey, a succulent roast, the perfect fish or vegetable dish —these make holiday dinners to remember all year.

ROAST TURKEY WITH FRUIT STUFFING

TURKEY
14-pound turkey
Salt and freshly ground black pepper

STUFFING
¼ pound butter or margarine
3 pounds tart cooking apples, peeled, cored, and sliced
⅔ cup coarsely chopped pitted prunes

GARNISH
6 slices of thick-cut bacon
1 pound link sausages

CRANBERRY GLAZE
1 cup cranberry sauce
2 teaspoons orange rind
2 tablespoons brown sugar, firmly packed
½ teaspoon ground ginger
2 tablespoons Worcestershire sauce
2 tablespoons water

1. Preheat oven to 375 degrees.
2. Remove giblets and set aside. Rinse turkey inside and out and pat dry. Season cavity with salt and pepper.
3. Make the stuffing: Melt half of the butter in a medium saucepan; add the apple pieces, cover the pan, shaking occasionally to keep apples from sticking. Cook gently until apples are tender. Stir in the prunes. When cool, spoon stuffing into turkey cavity.
4. Truss the turkey, then rub the outside with the remaining butter. Place turkey on a rack in a foil-lined roasting pan. Roast at 375 degrees for 15 minutes per pound. Then cook an additional 15 minutes more.
5. Make the garnish: Stretch each bacon slice with the back of a knife until double in length. Cut each into 2 or 3 strips, roll up and skewer. Place bacon rolls and sausages in the roasting pan the last half hour of cooking time and cook with the turkey.
6. Meanwhile, make the glaze: Blend all ingredients in medium saucepan. Bring to a boil, stirring constantly. Set aside.
7. Place turkey on serving platter, spoon glaze over turkey, and garnish with bacon and sausage. Serves 14 to 16.

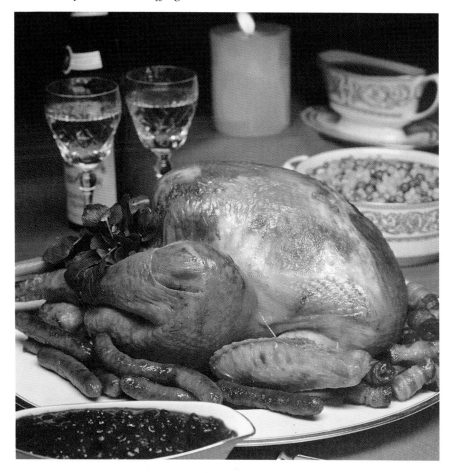

Roast Turkey with Fruit Stuffing

ROAST TURKEY	
Serving size:	3 ounces
Exchanges:	3 medium-fat meat
Calories:	225

FRUIT STUFFING	
Serving size:	½ cup
Exchanges:	2 fruit
	½ fat
Calories:	142

GARNISH	
Serving size:	1 ounce
Exchanges:	1 medium-fat meat
	2 fat
Calories:	165

CRANBERRY GLAZE	
Serving size:	Free

ROAST GOOSE WITH CHESTNUT-LIVER STUFFING

GOOSE
8- to 10-pound goose

STUFFING
2 pounds fresh chestnuts
2 cups chicken stock
2 tablespoons butter or margarine
6 large, tart cooking apples, peeled, cored, and sliced
2 large onions, peeled and chopped
2 cups bread crumbs
2 tablespoons chopped fresh parsley
1 tablespoon mixed dried thyme and marjoram
Grated rind of half a lemon
Salt and freshly ground black pepper

GRAVY
2 tablespoons flour
1 1/2 cups chicken stock or apple cider
2 tablespoons red currant jelly
Juice of half a lemon
Salt and freshly ground black pepper

1. Preheat oven to 400 degrees.
2. Remove giblet pack from goose, set aside. Remove liver and set goose aside.
3. Make the stuffing: Put chestnuts in boiling water. Cover and cook 5 to 6 minutes or until skins come off completely. Place chestnuts in stock and simmer until tender. Drain and let cool. Slice chestnuts in half and place pieces in large mixing bowl. Reserve stock for moistening the stuffing.
   Melt 1 tablespoon butter in medium skillet. Combine apples and

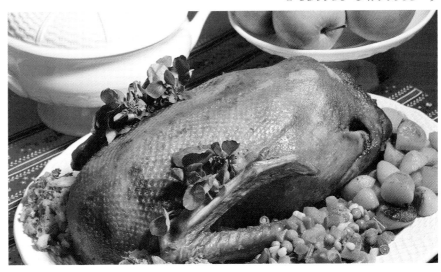

Roast Goose with Chestnut-Liver Stuffing

onions and saute 3 to 4 minutes over medium heat, or until tender. Combine with the chestnuts. Add remaining butter to skillet and saute the goose liver over medium heat. When firm, chop liver. Add with bread crumbs to the chestnut mixture.
   Add parsley, thyme and marjoram mixture, lemon rind, salt, and pepper. Mix together, adding enough stock to make moist but firm stuffing mixture.
4. Remove and discard loose fat in body cavity. Wash goose well and pat dry. Stuff neck cavity loosely; skewer shut. Spoon remaining stuffing into body cavity; skewer shut. Place the goose on a rack, breast side up, in a foil-lined roasting pan. Prick well on breast so fat will drain.
5. Roast at 400 degrees for 20 minutes, then reduce heat to 350 degrees and continue roasting for 20 to 25 minutes per pound, or until a meat thermometer inserted into the breast reads 185 degrees.
6. Remove goose from oven and place on serving platter; keep warm.

7. Make the gravy: Skim off 2 tablespoons fat from roasting pan. Put fat in saucepan. Whisk in flour. Blend in stock or cider, add red currant jelly and lemon juice, and stir well. Cook over low to medium heat, whisking constantly to avoid lumps and until mixture thickens. Season with salt and pepper to taste and serve hot with the goose. Serves 6 to 8.

ROAST GOOSE

Serving size:	3 ounces
Exchanges:	3 medium-fat meat
	1 fat
Calories:	270

CHESTNUT-LIVER STUFFING

Serving size:	1/2 cup
Exchanges:	2 medium-fat meat
	1 fruit
	2 fat
Calories:	300

GRAVY

Serving size:	1 ounce
Exchanges:	1/4 starch/bread
Calories:	20

DANISH CHRISTMAS DUCK

DUCK
5-pound duck
1 tablespoon butter
Salt and freshly ground black pepper

STUFFING
3 to 4 large cooking apples, peeled,
cored, and sliced
1 1/2 cups pitted prunes
Grated rind of half an orange
1/8 teaspoon each of salt and freshly
ground black pepper
2 cups chicken stock

GRAVY
1/4 cup port or red wine (optional)
1 tablespoon cornstarch
1 tablespoon cold water
1/4 cup heavy cream

1. Preheat oven to 350 degrees.
2. Rinse duck with cold water and pat dry. Prick breast with a fork to let fat drip. Rub skin with butter, salt, and pepper.
3. Prepare the stuffing: Mix apples and prunes together in large mixing bowl. Add orange rind, salt and pepper. Stir to combine. Spoon stuffing into duck cavity; skewer shut. Place duck on a rack, breast side up. Place rack on foil-lined roasting pan.
4. Roast at 350 degrees for 1 1/4 to 1 1/2 hours, basting frequently with pan drippings. Add 1 cup of stock to drippings halfway through cooking time. After 1 hour, skim fat off pan juices. Raise oven temperature to 400 degrees to brown duck well. Place duck on serving platter and keep hot.

5. Make the gravy: Skim remaining fat off drippings. Pour drippings into a medium saucepan. Add remaining stock. Cook over low heat for 3 to 4 minutes. Add port or red wine, if desired.

Mix cornstarch with 1 tablespoon cold water. Stir until mixture becomes a smooth paste. Spoon several tablespoons hot juice into cornstarch, stirring again. Slowly pour the cornstarch mixture into the gravy, and stir constantly until mixture thickens. Add cream; serve gravy hot with duck. Serves 4 to 6.

DANISH CHRISTMAS DUCK

Serving size:	3 ounces
Exchanges:	3 medium-fat meat
	1 fat
Calories:	270

STUFFING

Serving size:	1/2 cup
Exchanges:	2 starch/bread
Calories:	160

GRAVY

Serving size:	1 ounce
Exchanges:	1 fat
Calories:	45

ROAST DUCK WITH APRICOT STUFFING

DUCK
4- to 5-pound duck
3 tablespoons honey

STUFFING
1 large orange

16-ounce can halved apricots, drained, or
1 pound fresh apricots, peeled and pitted
1 large onion, peeled and diced
Salt and freshly ground black pepper

SAUCE
1 to 1 1/2 cups chicken stock
3 to 4 tablespoons apricot brandy

1. Preheat oven to 400 degrees.
2. Remove giblets; set aside for another use. Rinse and drain duck and pat dry.

With a sharp paring knife, peel the thin outer skin, or zest, from orange into 3 long, narrow strips. Set orange aside. Combine zest in mixing bowl with half the apricots, onion, salt, and pepper. Spoon this stuffing into duck cavity. Prick skin all over so fat will drain. Season skin with salt and pepper. Place duck on rack in foil-lined roasting pan. Roast at 400 degrees for 20 minutes per pound.
3. Meanwhile, warm honey in saucepan and stir in juice from orange. Half an hour before end of cooking time, spoon honey mixture over duck. Ten minutes before end of cooking time, add apricots to pan to brown.
4. When duck is done, remove from oven and put on serving platter. Garnish with apricots. Keep warm.
5. Make the sauce: Remove stuffing and place in large saucepan. Skim fat off drippings and pour drippings into saucepan with stuffing. Add stock and bring to a boil, stirring constantly. After 5 minutes, pour mixture into container of blender or food processor and blend. Return to saucepan, add brandy, and heat. Serves 4 to 6.

ROAST DUCK

Serving size:	3 ounces
Exchanges:	3 medium-fat meat
	1 fat
Calories:	270

APRICOT STUFFING

Serving size:	¹/2 cup
Exchanges:	1 starch/bread
	1 fruit
Calories:	140

WILD DUCK WITH RED CABBAGE

CABBAGE

3 large onions, peeled and chopped
1¹/2-pound head red cabbage, cored and
shredded finely
2 to 3 tablespoons red wine vinegar
2 to 3 tablespoons water
Salt and freshly ground black pepper
4 tart cooking apples, peeled, cored, and
sliced
1 teaspoon sugar

DUCK

3 tablespoons vegetable oil
2- to 3-pound duck, preferably wild,
cut into quarters
1 teaspoon caraway seeds
¹/2 cup chicken stock
1 tablespoon chopped parsley

1. Preheat oven to 350 degrees.
2. Grease a 2-quart baking dish. Prepare cabbage: Mix onions with cabbage and place in dish. Add vinegar, water, salt, and pepper. Cover tightly and bake for 1 hour. Add sliced apples and sugar. Cook for 15 minutes more.

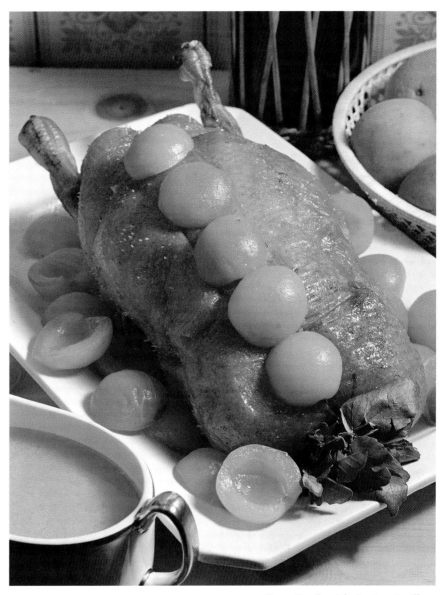

Roast Duck with Apricot Stuffing

3. Heat oil in a heavy skillet. When hot, brown pieces of duck. Remove duck pieces and place on cabbage in casserole. Sprinkle with caraway seeds and add the stock. Cover and bake for 30 to 40 minutes, or until tender.
4. Sprinkle with chopped parsley. Serve hot. Serves 4 to 6.

WILD DUCK

Serving size:	3 ounces
Exchanges:	3 medium-fat meat
	1 fat
Calories:	270

RED CABBAGE

Serving size:	¹/2 cup
Exchanges:	1 starch/bread
	2 fruit
Calories:	200

SQUABS STUFFED WITH RAISINS AND ALMONDS

STUFFING
1/4 cup raisins
2 to 3 tablespoons dry sherry
3 tablespoons butter or margarine
2 large onions, peeled and chopped
1 cup cooked long-grain white rice
3 to 4 tablespoons slivered almonds
1 tablespoon chopped fresh mixed thyme and marjoram, or 1 teaspoon dried

SQUABS
4 squabs (1 pound each)
4 slices thick-cut bacon
2 to 3 tablespoons vegetable oil
1 to 2 teaspoons flour
1/2 cup red wine
1/2 cup chicken stock
Salt and freshly ground black pepper

1. Preheat oven to 400 degrees. Soak raisins in sherry and set aside.
2. Make the stuffing: Melt butter in skillet and saute onions until soft and golden. Add cooked rice and saute for 1 minute. Add almonds, herbs, and raisins. Stir to combine. Spoon stuffing into body cavity.
3. Skewer a slice of bacon around breast of each bird. Pour oil into large roasting pan and heat. Place squabs in pan and baste thoroughly.
4. Roast for about 35 to 40 minutes, basting and turning every 10 minutes. Remove bacon for last 15 minutes to brown breasts. Remove squabs from oven. Place on serving platter; keep warm.
5. Make the gravy: Skim oil off drippings. Pour drippings into medium saucepan. Sprinkle and blend flour into drippings. Add wine and stock. Cook over low heat, stirring until smooth. Season with salt and pepper. Serve with squabs. Serves 4.

SQUAB	
Serving size:	3 ounces
Exchanges:	3 medium-fat meat
Calories:	225

STUFFING	
Serving size:	1/2 cup
Exchanges:	1 starch/bread
	1 fat
Calories:	125

GRAVY	
Serving size:	1 ounces
Exchanges:	1 fat
Calories:	45

ROCK CORNISH GAME HENS WITH MINCEMEAT STUFFING

CORNISH HENS
2 Rock Cornish game hens (1 1/2 pounds each)
1/4 cup butter, melted

STUFFING
4 slices whole-wheat bread, cubed
3/4 cup orange juice
1/2 cup prepared mincemeat, drained
1/4 cup diced celery
1/2 teaspoon salt

1. Preheat oven to 375 degrees.
2. Remove giblets and necks from hens and discard. Rinse and drain hens and pat dry. Truss hens securely. Place them breast side up on rack in a foil-lined roasting pan.
3. Roast for 1 to 1 1/2 hours, brushing every 15 minutes with melted butter.
4. Make the stuffing: Combine in a 1-quart baking dish the bread cubes, orange juice, mincemeat, celery, and salt. Put in baking dish and bake stuffing with hens for the last 30 minutes of roasting time.
5. Place hens and stuffing on serving platter. Serves 4.

ROCK CORNISH GAME HENS	
Serving size:	3 ounces
Exchanges:	3 medium-fat meat
Calories:	225

STUFFING	
Serving size:	1/2 cup
Exchanges:	1/2 starch/bread
Calories:	40

FRESH GAME BIRD PIE

PASTRY
1 cup flour
1/8 teaspoon salt
1/2 cup water
1/2 cup butter
2 large eggs
1/4 cup grated Cheddar cheese
1/2 teaspoon dried mustard

FILLING
2 tablespoons butter or margarine
1 large onion, peeled and chopped
6 to 8 large mushrooms, sliced
1 tablespoon flour
1 teaspoon tomato paste
1/2 cup chicken stock
2 tablespoons dry sherry

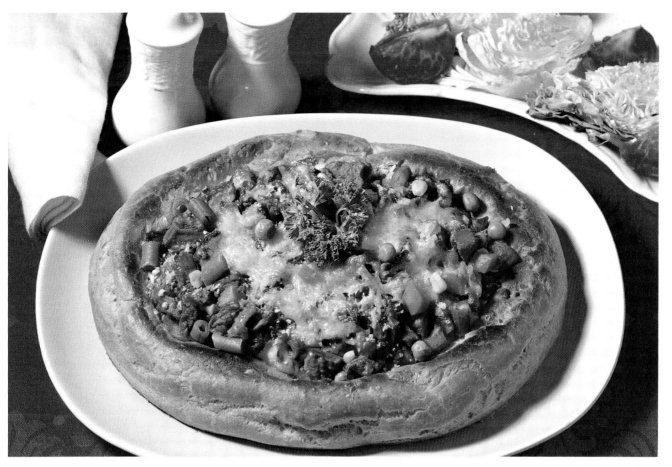

Fresh Game Bird Pie

1 cup cooked and cubed grouse and
partridge, or other game
$^1/_2$ tablespoon chopped fresh thyme
$^1/_2$ tablespoon fresh chopped parsley, or
1 teaspoon each dried
$^1/_2$ cup cooked, cubed vegetables,
as available
1 teaspoon Worcestershire sauce
3 tablespoons freshly grated Parmesan
cheese
2 tablespoons white bread crumbs
1 tablespoon chopped fresh parsley

1. Preheat oven to 375 degrees.
2. Make the pastry: Sift flour with salt into large mixing bowl; set aside. In a medium saucepan, heat $^1/_2$ cup water and butter. When butter melts, bring mixture to a boil.

Remove from heat and add flour all at once. Beat with spoon until mixture forms a ball in bottom of pan. Spread out on a plate to cool. Place cooled flour mixture in a mixing bow. Beat eggs and add to flour mixture gradually, beating constantly between each addition. The mixture should be shiny, smooth and hold its shape. Some egg may be left over; discard. Add cheese and dried mustard; set aside.

3. Make the filling: Melt butter in large saucepan, add onion, and cook 5 to 6 minutes or until soft. Add mushrooms; cook for 1 minute. Sprinkle and stir in flour; add tomato paste and stock. Bring mixture to a boil. Cook, stirring constantly, until it thickens.

Remove from heat. Add sherry, meat, herbs, vegetables, and Worcestershire sauce. Let cool slightly.

4. Grease 2-quart baking dish at least 3 inches deep. Press dough onto bottom and sides of dish and brush with any remaining egg. Spoon filling into center of pastry ring. Sprinkle top with cheese, bread crumbs, and parsley. Bake at 375 degrees for 30 to 45 minutes. Remove from oven. Serves 4.

Serving size:	6 ounces
Exchanges:	1 starch/bread
	1 medium-fat meat
	1 fruit
	1 fat
Calories:	260

ROAST CAPON WITH ORANGE PECAN STUFFING

STUFFING

1/4 cup butter or margarine
1 cup thinly sliced celery
1/4 cup chopped onion
3/4 cup water
5 cups of 1/2-inch-thick toasted, crustless bread cubes
3/4 cups sectioned and diced orange
1/6 cup coarsely chopped pecans
1 teaspoon grated orange rind
1 teaspoon salt
1/2 teaspoon curry powder (optional)

ROAST CAPON

5- to 6-pound capon
Melted butter for brushing on skin
Orange slices and watercress for garnish

1. Preheat oven to 325 degrees.
2. Make the stuffing: Melt butter in a medium skillet. Add the celery, onion, and water. Cook over medium heat until the vegetables are tender. Combine the bread cubes, orange, pecans, orange rind, 1/2 teaspoon salt, and curry powder in a mixing bowl. Mix together, stir in vegetables.
3. Rinse the capon and pat dry. Sprinkle the remaining salt in the neck and body cavities. Spoon stuffing loosely into neck and body cavities. Skewer the neck skin to back and tuck legs and wings close to body. Put capon, breast side up, on a rack in a foil-lined roasting pan. Brush the skin with butter. Cover the capon loosely with foil, crimping it to the edges of the pan. Foil should not touch capon.

4. Roast for about 3 hours. Remove the foil 45 minutes before end of cooking time to allow the bird to brown. Brush with melted butter.
5. Place capon on serving platter and garnish. Serves 6 to 8.

ROAST CAPON

Serving size:	3 ounces
Exchanges:	3 medium-fat meat
Calories:	225

STUFFING

Serving size:	1/2 cup
Exchanges:	1 1/2 starch/bread
	4 fat
Calories:	300

ORANGE-BAKED CHICKEN

2-pound roasting chicken
2 tablespoons chopped onions
1/2 teaspoon paprika
1/4 teaspoon rosemary
1/4 teaspoon salt
1/4 teaspoon black pepper
1 cup orange juice
4 small carrots, peeled and sliced

1. Preheat oven to 300 degrees.
2. Place chicken in ovenproof casserole. Sprinkle with onions, paprika, rosemary, salt, and pepper. Bake, basting frequently with orange juice about 2 hours, or until chicken is brown and tender.
3. Steam fresh carrots; brown in pan juices from the chicken.
4. Place chicken on serving platter. Spoon carrots around chicken. Serves 4.

Serving size:	3 ounces
Exchanges:	3 medium-fat meat
	1 fruit
Calories:	285

FRENCH HERBED CHICKEN

3-pound broiler/fryer chicken, cut up
1 tablespoon shortening
Salt and freshly ground black pepper
8-ounce can small whole onions, drained
1/2 cup coarsely chopped carrots
1 garlic clove, crushed
2 tablespoons snipped parsley
1/2 teaspoon dried thyme, crushed
2-ounce can sliced mushrooms
1 cup sauterne
2 to 3 stalks celery, cut up
1 medium bay leaf

1. Preheat oven to 350 degrees.
2. In skillet, brown chicken in hot fat. Season with salt and pepper and place in 2-quart casserole.
3. Drain excess fat in skillet. Add remaining ingredients except celery and bay leaf. Heat, scraping up browned pieces.
4. Pour over chicken. Tuck in celery and bay leaf. Cover and bake at 350 degrees for 1 1/4 hours. Remove bay leaf and celery.
5. Place chicken on serving platter. Serves 4.

Serving size:	3 ounces
Exchanges:	3 lean meat
	1 vegetable
Calories:	190

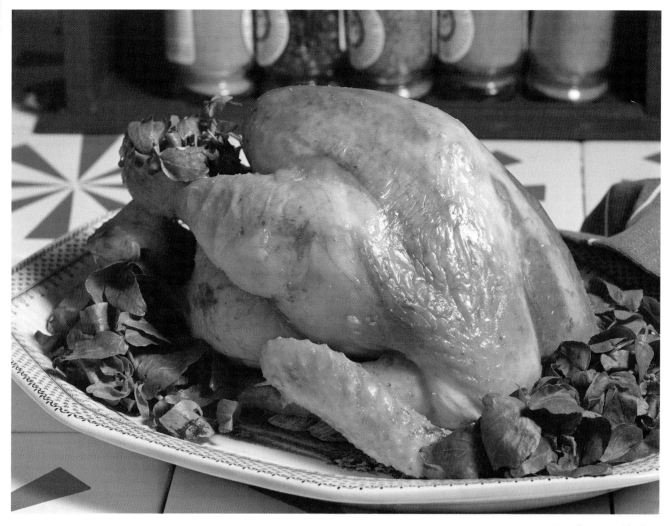

French Roast Chicken

FRENCH ROAST CHICKEN

3- to 4-pound roasting chicken
1 large onion, peeled and diced
1 teaspoon poultry seasoning
1¹/₂ cups water
6 to 7 tablespoons butter or margarine
3 to 4 sprigs chopped fresh parsley
Salt and freshly ground black pepper
3 slices bacon
1 bunch watercress

1. Preheat oven to 350 degrees.
2. Make the stock: Remove giblets from chicken and combine them with onion, poultry seasoning, and water in a saucepan. Simmer for 15 minutes.
3. Meanwhile, put half of the butter and the parsley, salt, and pepper into cavity of the chicken. Rub the remaining butter on the skin. Cover the breast with bacon slices. Place chicken, breast side down, on rack in foil-lined roasting pan.
4. Roast for 20 minutes per pound. Baste chicken with stock every 15 minutes. For the last 20 minutes, remove bacon slices, turn chicken, breast side up, to brown, and brush with pan drippings.
5. Place chicken on serving platter. Skim fat off drippings. Pour drippings into saucepan with remaining stock. Boil for three minutes to reduce, then serve as gravy.
6. At serving time, garnish chicken with sprigs of watercress. Offer guests a side salad of watercress dressed with a mild vinaigrette. Serves 4 to 6.

Serving size:	3 ounces
Exchanges:	3 medium-fat meat
Calories:	225

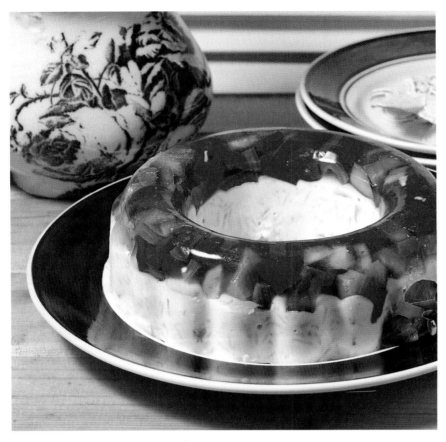

Molded Chicken Salad

Serving size:	1 cup
Exchanges:	1 starch/bread
	3 medium-fat meat
Calories:	305

BEEF TENDERLOIN FILLETS

2 1/2 pounds beef tenderloin
1 cup plus 2 tablespoons butter or margarine
2 tablespoons chopped onion
1 slice thick-cut bacon, diced
1/2 tablespoon flour
1 teaspoon tomato puree
8 large mushrooms, stems and caps separated, stems chopped
2 cups beef stock
1/4 cup red wine
Salt and freshly ground black pepper
1 tablespoon fresh chopped mixed parsley and thyme, or 1 teaspoon each of the dried
8 slices white bread
1 cup vegetable oil
8-ounce can duck pate
Watercress for garnish

MOLDED CHICKEN SALAD

1 envelope unflavored gelatin
1/4 cup cold water
1 cup hot chicken stock
2 tablespoons chopped red pepper
2 tablespoons chopped green pepper
2 cups diced cooked chicken
1 tablespoon finely chopped onion
1 cup chopped celery
1 cup cooked rice
1/2 teaspoon salt
1/4 cup French dressing
1/8 teaspoon paprika
1/2 cup mayonnaise
Lettuce

1. Combine the gelatin and cold water and leave for about 10 minutes to soften. Add hot chicken stock and stir until the gelatin has melted.

2. Rinse a 6-cup mold with cold water, then add the red and green peppers. Cover with 2 tablespoons of the melted gelatin and refrigerate until set.

3. Mix all the ingredients except the lettuce. Add the remaining gelatin.

4. When the gelatin in the mold is quite firm, spoon the chicken mixture on top. Leave until set.

5. Unmold and serve on a bed of lettuce. Serves 6.

1. Preheat the oven to 350 degrees.

2. Cut tenderloin into 1/2-inch thick slices. Make the sauce: Melt 1 tablespoon butter or margarine in a saucepan. Add onion and bacon; cook slowly and stir until golden. Stir in flour and cook mixture until light brown. Add tomato puree, mushroom stems, stock, wine, salt, and pepper. Bring to a boil, then reduce heat and simmer for 15 minutes. Add parsley-thyme mixture and simmer 4 or 5 more minutes. Strain through a fine sieve into a serving dish; keep warm.

3. Butter a 9 x 12-inch baking dish and place mushroom caps in it. Cut 1 tablespoon butter into 8 pieces; dot each cap with butter. Sprinkle caps with salt and pepper to taste. Bake for 10 minutes. Keep warm.

4. Meanwhile, trim bread to fit fillet slices. Heat oil and 1 tablespoon butter in skillet. When butter foams, fry bread until golden on each side. Drain on paper towels and keep warm.

5. In another skillet, melt remaining butter. When it foams, saute the fillets for 4 to 6 minutes on each side. Arrange bread on a serving platter. Open can of pate and slice into 8 equal pieces. Place 1 fillet on each slice of fried bread. Top each with a slice of pate and a mushroom cap. Spoon sauce over top. Garnish platter with watercress. Serves 8.

Serving size:	1 fillet
Exchanges:	1 starch/bread
	5 medium-fat meat
	1 vegetable
	4 fat
Calories:	660

STANDING RIB ROAST

3-rib standing rib roast, about
8 pounds
Salt and freshly ground black pepper

1. Preheat oven to 400 degrees.
2. Stand the roast, fat side up, on a rack in a foil-lined roasting pan. Add no water. Insert a meat thermometer into the center of the roast, making sure point rests on meat.

3. Roast uncovered at 400 degrees for 15 minutes. Lower temperature to 375. Roast until thermometer reads 140 degrees for rare (about 23 to 25 minutes per pound), 160 degrees for medium (about 27 to 30 minutes per pound), and 170 degrees for well done (about 32 to 35 minutes per pound).

4. Place roast on warm serving platter. Season with salt and pepper and slice. Serves 8 to 10.

Serving size:	3 ounces no bone
Exchanges:	3 medium-fat meat
	1 fat
Calories:	270

Beef Tenderloin Fillets

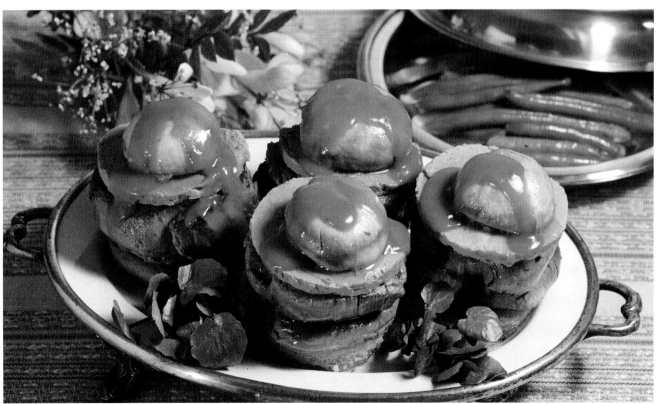

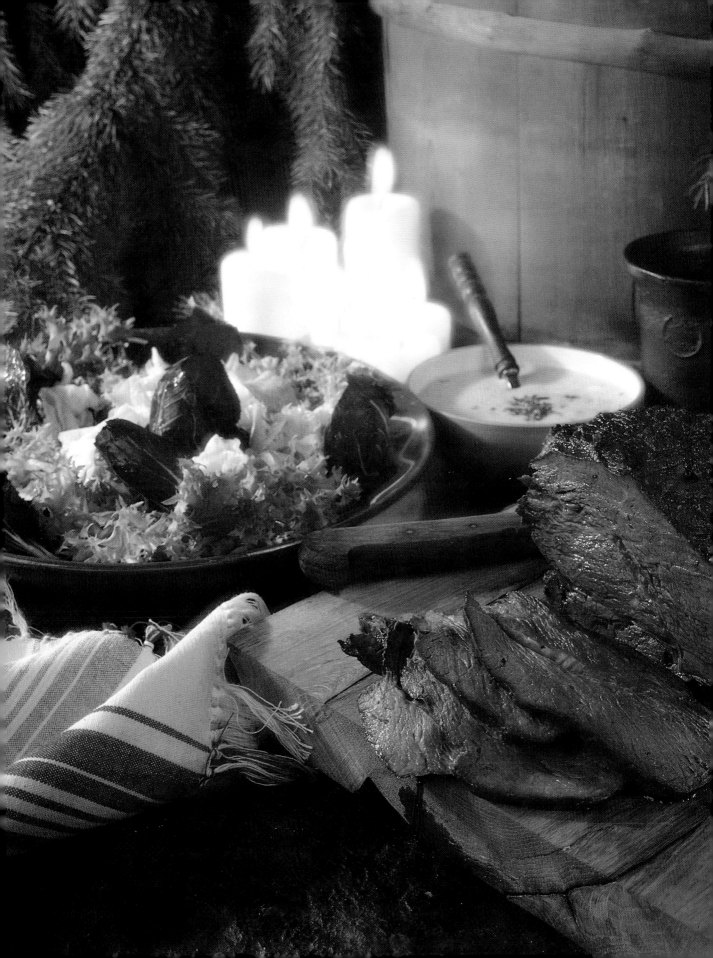

ROAST BEEF WITH NOBIS SAUCE

ROAST BEEF
3³/₄ pounds boneless roast beef
2¹/₂ teaspoons salt
¹/₂ to 1 teaspoon freshly ground black pepper

NOBIS SAUCE
1 large egg
2¹/₂ to 3 teaspoons white wine vinegar
³/₄ cup extra-virgin olive oil
Salt and freshly ground black pepper
1 teaspoon Dijon-style mustard
1 tablespoon snipped chives
1 garlic clove, mashed

1. Preheat oven to 375 degrees.
2. Season the meat on all sides with salt and pepper. Insert a meat thermometer into the roast until tip of the thermometer reaches the center of the roast. Place the roast in a foil-lined roasting pan. Then place pan in oven. Roast at 375 degrees for 1 to 1¹/₄ hours or until the thermometer reads 140 degrees for rare, 160 degrees for medium, or 170 degrees for well done.
3. Make the sauce: Place egg in boiling water to cover. Boil for exactly 3 minutes. Remove egg from heat. Break open and spoon out the insides into a mixing bowl. Alternate adding drops of vinegar and oil, whisking constantly after each addition. The sauce should thicken to the consistency of mayonnaise. Season with salt and pepper to taste. Stir in mustard, chives, and garlic. Refrigerate before serving.

Roast Beef with Nobis Sauce

4. Place roast on serving platter. Serve with chilled sauce.
Serves 6 to 8.

ROAST BEEF	
Serving size:	3 ounces
Exchanges:	3 medium-fat meat
Calories:	225

NOBIS SAUCE	
Serving size:	1 ounce
Exchanges:	2 fat
Calories:	90

PORK ROAST WITH CRANBERRY STUFFING

PORK
6- to 7-pound pork loin roast (with backbone removed)
Salt and freshly ground black pepper
1 teaspoon poultry seasoning

STUFFING
1 cup boiling beef broth
¹/₂ cup butter or margarine
8-ounce package herb-seasoned bread stuffing
1 cup coarsely chopped fresh cranberries
1 small tart red apple, unpeeled, cored, and diced
¹/₄ cup finely chopped celery
¹/₄ cup minced parsley
1 large egg
Parsley sprigs and sliced oranges for garnish

1. Preheat oven to 350 degrees.
2. Place the roast, rib ends up, on a cutting board. Hold the meaty side of the roast with one hand. Start 1 inch from end of roast and slit a

pocket between the meat and rib bones almost to the bottom of the roast. Finish 1 inch from the other end. Pull the meaty part slightly away from the ribs to open the pocket. Sprinkle the inside of the pocket with salt, pepper, and poultry seasoning.
3. Make the stuffing: Pour boiling broth into a medium saucepan and add butter. Over low heat, melt butter, stirring mixture occasionally.
4. Remove from heat. Add the bread stuffing, cranberries, apple, celery, and parsley. Mix well.
5. Beat the egg until thick and pale. Mix with the stuffing, then spoon mixture into pocket. Spoon any extra stuffing into a small baking dish and set aside. Place pork on rack in foil-lined roasting pan.
6. Roast at 350 degrees for 35 minutes per pound. About half an hour before roast should be ready, place baking dish with extra stuffing in the oven.
7. Place roast on hot serving platter. Skim fat off drippings. Then spoon drippings over stuffing in pocket and in baking dish. Serve immediately. Use parsley sprigs and sliced oranges for garnish. Serves 6.

ROAST PORK	
Serving size:	3 ounces
Exchanges:	3 medium-fat meat
	2 fat
Calories:	315

STUFFING	
Serving size:	¹/₂ cup
Exchanges:	1 starch/bread
	1 fruit
	2 fat
Calories:	230

CROWN ROAST OF PORK WITH ORANGE RICE

PORK
2 pieces of pork loin roast
(6 ribs each)
Salt and freshly ground black pepper

ORANGE RICE
¼ cup butter or margarine
1 cup finely chopped celery
1 large onion, peeled and chopped
1 pound uncooked long-grain white rice
2 teaspoons salt
2½ cups chicken stock
1 cup orange juice
½ cup raisins
1 tablespoon grated orange rind
Grapes and watercress for garnish

1. Ask butcher to prepare meat for a crown roast.
2. Preheat oven to 350 degrees.

Crown Roast of Pork with Orange Rice

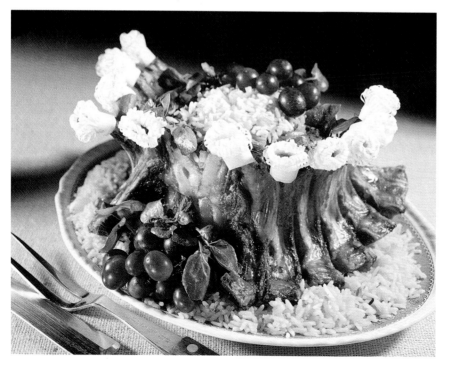

3. Form loins into a circle. Sew together with fine string and tie a double length of string around roast to hold shape. Wrap bone ends in foil. Sprinkle pork with salt and pepper and place in foil-lined roasting pan. Roast at 350 degrees for 30 minutes per pound, plus 30 minutes more.

4. Make the orange rice: Heat butter in large saucepan. Stir in celery, onion, rice, and salt. Add stock and orange juice; bring to a boil. Stir, then cover pan. Simmer gently for 15 minutes, or until rice is tender and all liquid is absorbed. Stir in raisins and orange rind.

5. Place roast on serving platter. Spoon rice stuffing in towel in center; serve extra rice stuffing in separate serving dish. Remove foil from bones. Garnish platter with grapes and watercress. Serves 10 to 12.

NOTE: Use brown or Indian Basmati rice instead of standard white rice for a change of pace.

CROWN ROAST OF PORK	
Serving size:	3 ounces
Exchanges:	3 medium-fat meat
	2 fat
Calories:	310

ORANGE RICE	
Serving size:	½ cup
Exchanges:	1 starch/bread
Calories:	80

SAVORY PORK IN SWEET POTATO NESTS

2 cups mashed sweet potatoes
½ to 1 cup milk
1 tablespoon melted butter
or margarine
1½ cups cooked pork, finely chopped
1 cup peas
½ cup pork or other gravy
Salt and freshly ground black pepper
¼ teaspoon dried thyme

1. Preheat oven to 350 degrees.
2. Place mashed sweet potatoes in a mixing bowl. Add enough milk to make a smooth, easy-to-shape mixture. Scoop 4 equal mounds onto baking sheet. Make a well in the center of each mound with the back of a spoon. Brush with melted butter.
3. Combine remaining ingredients in a baking dish. Bake the pork mixture and sweet potato mounds for 15 to 20 minutes. When ready to serve, spoon pork mixture into the sweet potato nests. Serves 4.

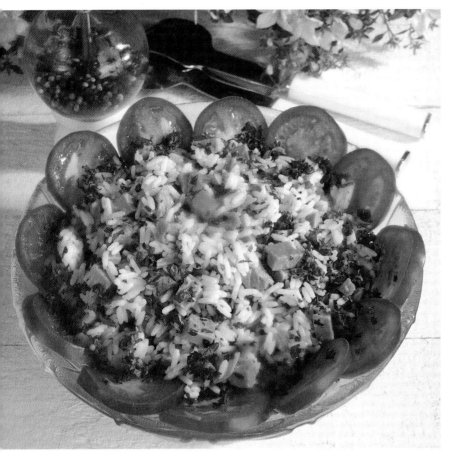

Rice Salad with Ham

Serving size:	1 Nest
Exchanges:	3 starch/bread
	3 medium-fat meat
	1 fruit
	3 fat
Calories:	660

SOUTHAMPTON HAM

10- to 12-pound Smithfield or Virginia country ham
6 to 7 cups cold water, or 5 1/2 cups cold water plus 1 1/2 cups dry sherry

1. Soak the ham overnight or for about 8 hours in water to cover.
2. Preheat oven to 500 degrees.

Rinse the ham under running water and scrub off its pepper coating with a stiff brush. Place ham in a roaster and add water or water and sherry. Place a tightly fitting lid on the roaster, making sure any vents are closed. Bake ham for 15 to 20 minutes. Turn off the oven. Keep oven door shut for the entire cooking time of ham.

3. Keep ham in oven for 3 hours. Turn heat back on to 500 degrees and cook ham for another 20 minutes. At this time, the rind and excess fat can be cut away and the ham glazed, if desired. Turn heat off again. Allow ham to remain in the oven undisturbed for another 3 hours or

overnight. Slice ham wafer thin. Do not use this cooking process on hams over 12 pounds.

4. To prepare the ham in one day: Soak the ham in the early morning. About 6:00 p.m., begin the first phase of cooking. At about 9:30, turn the heat back on to complete the cooking. Turn off the oven and leave the ham undisturbed until the next morning. Serves 18 to 20.

Serving size:	3 ounces
Exchanges:	3 medium-fat meat
Calories:	225

RICE SALAD WITH HAM

2/3 cup rice
1 1/2 tablespoons vinegar
1/2 teaspoon salt
1/4 teaspoon black or white pepper
1 garlic clove, crushed
1 teaspoon tarragon (optional)
3 tablespoons oil
2 tablespoons water
1 pound ham, cut into cubes
1/4 cup parsley, finely chopped

1. Boil the rice according to the directions given on the package.
2. Mix together the vinegar, spices, oil, and water. Pour the dressing over the hot rice. Let stand until the rice becomes cold.
3. Mix the cold rice with the ham and parsley. Serves 4.

Serving size:	4 ounces
Exchanges:	1/2 starch/bread
	3 medium-fat meat
Calories:	265

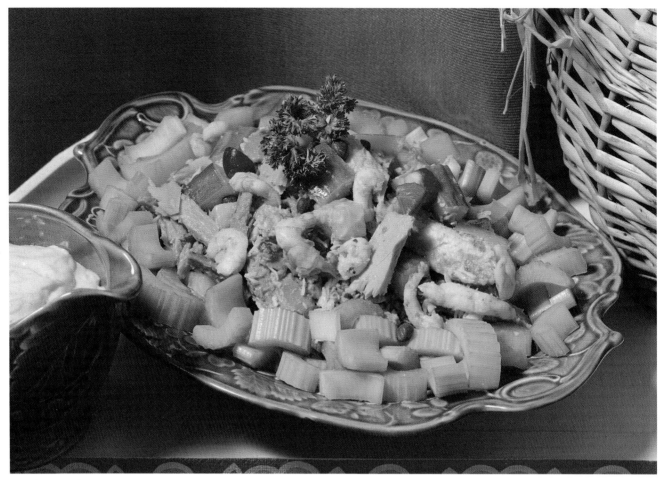

Seafood Medley

PINEAPPLE-GLAZED BAKED HAM

3- to 5-pound fully cooked, cured ham
Whole cloves
8-ounce can juice-packed pineapple rings
6-ounce can pineapple juice concentrate, defrosted, undiluted
2 teaspoons prepared mustard

1. Preheat oven to 325 degrees.
2. Place ham, fat side up, on a rack in a roasting pan. Insert meat thermometer in thickest part, not touching bone. Bake, uncovered, no water added, for about 20 minutes per pound. After 45 to 60 minutes, remove from oven. Drain and discard melted fat in the pan.
3. With a sharp knife, trim away most of the skin and fat from the ham. Score surface into a diamond pattern and decorate with whole cloves. Arrange pineapple rings on top of ham, secure with toothpicks or cloves. Combine remaining ingredients (including juice from rings) and pour over ham.
4. Return to the oven. Continue to bake, basting often, until thermometer reads 140 degrees.
5. Remove from oven to a cutting board. Wait 15 minutes before carving. Skim fat from pan juices and use as a sauce. Serves 12.

Serving size:	3 ounces
Exchanges:	3 medium-fat meat
	1/2 fruit
Calories:	255

HAM STEAK WITH PINEAPPLE RAISIN SAUCE

1 1/4 pounds ready-to-eat ham steak
1/2 cup unsweetened pineapple juice
1/8 teaspoon ground cloves
1/8 teaspoon ground cinnamon
3 tablespoons white (golden) raisins

1. Trim fringe fat from ham steak.
2. Spray a nonstick skillet with

cooking spray. Brown the ham steak in the skillet about 3 to 4 minutes on each side. Remove to a platter.

3. Combine remaining ingredients in skillet over high heat. Cook and stir minute. Pour over ham. Serves 4.

Serving size:	5 ounces
Exchanges:	5 medium-fat meat
	1/2 fruit
Calories:	405

SEAFOOD MEDLEY

6 1/2-ounce can tuna fish
6 1/2-ounce can crabmeat
4 1/4-ounce can shrimp
1/2 cup French dressing
1 cup diced celery
1/2 cup diced cucumber
6 to 8 radishes, chopped
1 tablespoon capers
2 tablespoons lemon juice
1/2 cup mayonnaise
Salt and freshly ground black pepper
Paprika to taste
Lettuce

1. Drain the tuna and break up into flakes. Add flaked crabmeat and shrimp. Stir in the French dressing. Set aside to chill for about 15 minutes.

2. Add celery, cucumber, radishes, and capers.

3. Blend lemon juice with the mayonnaise, add seasoning to taste. Toss all ingredients lightly together.

4. Serve on on top of crisp lettuce. Serves 5 to 6.

Serving size:	4 ounces
Exchanges:	4 lean meat
	2 fat
Calories:	310

STUFFED PEPPERS

GARNISH
6 slices thick-cut bacon
parsley for garnish

SAUCE
3 tablespoons butter or margarine
3 tablespoons flour
1 1/2 cups grated Cheddar cheese
1/2 to 1 cup beer or ale
Salt and freshly ground black pepper
Dash of hot pepper sauce

PEPPERS
4 large green bell peppers, tops and seeds removed
4 cups cooked long-grain white rice
4 hard-boiled eggs, peeled and minced

1. Place strips of bacon in a large skillet and cook until crisp. Remove from skillet, drain on paper towel, and crumble. Set aside for use as a garnish.

2. Make the sauce: Place butter in a large saucepan. Heat until melted. Stir in the flour, and add the cheese, beer, and seasonings. Stir until the sauce thickens.

3. Slice off the rounded bottoms of the peppers so they will stand upright. Place peppers in a baking dish. Add the rice and eggs to the cheese mixture, stirring to combine. Spoon mixture into each hollow pepper. Sprinkle tops with crumbled bacon. Garnish with sprigs of parsley,

if desired. Wrap in foil and serve. Serves 4.

Serving size:	1 serving
Exchanges:	4 starch/bread
	1 medium-fat meat
	1 fruit
	4 fat
Calories:	635

FLOUNDER ITALIANO

1 teaspoon salt
4 4-ounce halibut steaks
3/4 cup chicken bouillon
1/4 cup wine vinegar
2 tablespoons finely chopped parsley
1 small garlic clove, minced
1/2 teaspoon oregano leaves
Fresh dill and lemon wedges for garnish
Paprika

1. Sprinkle salt on the steaks, then place them in a large shallow pan. Combine bouillon, vinegar, parsley, garlic, and oregano in small bowl and pour over fish. Then marinate in refrigerator for two hours.

2. Preheat broiler.

3. Place steaks on a rack on broiling pan about 4 inches from heat. Broil for 8 minutes or until fish flakes easily with a fork. Baste with marinade several times during broiling, turning once.

4. Arrange on serving platter. Garnish with dill and lemon wedges; sprinkle with paprika. Serves 4.

Serving size:	4 ounces
Exchanges:	4 lean meat
Calories:	220

SHRIMP MARENGO

*1/2 pound raw, unpeeled **jumbo** shrimp,
fresh or defrosted*
1 teaspoon olive oil
*2 tablespoons olive juice, from jar of
olives*
1 garlic clove, minced
1 large sweet Spanish onion, chopped
*2 vine-ripe tomatoes, peeled and diced
(or 8-ounce can tomatoes)*
1 cup tomato juice
1/4 cup dry white wine
1/4 cup chopped fresh parsley
1/4 teaspoon dried basil or oregano
6 pitted ripe olives, sliced thin
1 lemon, cut in wedges, for garnish

1. Peel raw shrimp and set aside.
2. Combine olive oil, olive juice,
and garlic in a large nonstick skillet
sprayed with cooking spray. Cook,
uncovered, over moderate heat until
liquid evaporates. Add onion; cook
and stir 2 minutes, but do not
brown. Stir in tomatoes, tomato
juice, wine, parsley, basil or oregano,
and olives. Lower heat and simmer,
uncovered, 5 minutes.
3. Arrange peeled raw shrimp on
top of mixture. Simmer, uncovered, 1
to 2 minutes. Turn shrimp and continue to simmer an additional 1 or 2
minutes. Shrimp should be pink and
cooked through and liquid evaporated into a thick sauce. Garnish with
lemon, if desired. Serves 2.

Serving size:	1 serving
Exchanges:	1 starch/bread
	3 lean meat
Calories:	245

FILLETS OF SOLE IN MUSHROOM SAUCE

MUSHROOM SAUCE
1/2 pound fresh mushrooms, thinly sliced
1/4 cup minced onion or scallion
*3 tablespoons dry sherry or other white
wine*
1 tablespoon butter or margarine
1 cup skim milk
2 tablespoons instant-blending flour

FISH FILLETS
*2 pounds sole or flounder fillets, fresh or
defrosted*
Salt and freshly ground black pepper
Paprika to taste
1 tablespoon chopped fresh parsley

1. Prepare sauce: Combine mushrooms, onion, sherry, and butter in a
large nonstick skillet or electric frying
pan sprayed with cooking spray. Cook
and stir over moderate heat until wine
evaporates and mushrooms begin to
brown. Lower heat.
2. Combine milk and flour and
stir until smooth. Stir into skillet
until mixture simmers and thickens.
3. Arrange fish fillets in skillet on
top of sauce. Sprinkle fish lightly
with salt, pepper, and paprika. Cover
skillet; simmer over very low heat
until fish flakes easily, about 10 to 12
minutes. Gently transfer fillets to a
hot platter. Stir parsley into skillet
sauce. Spoon sauce over fish and
serve immediately. Serves 8.

Serving size:	2 ounces
Exchanges:	1/2 starch/bread
	2 lean meat
Calories:	150

QUICK PAELLA

1 pound white fish, fresh or frozen
1 onion, peeled and chopped
2 tablespoons margarine
*1 teaspoon curry powder or 1/2 envelope
saffron*
1 cup long-grain rice
2 cups chicken broth
1 1/2 teaspoons salt
1 cup frozen peas
1/2 cup chopped red pepper
1 1/4 cups fresh shrimp in shells
Lemon wedges for garnish

1. If the fish is frozen, place it in
lukewarm water.
2. In a wide frying pan, saute the
onion in the margarine until transparent. Dust the onion with curry
powder or saffron. Add the rice and
the chicken broth. Cover the pan and
simmer for 10 minutes.
3. Cut the fish into 2-inch pieces;
season with salt. Press them into the
rice, which will have expanded and
absorbed most of the liquid. Place
the peas, red pepper, and shrimp on
top of the rice. Cover and cook for
10 more minutes.
4. Serve in the pan or in a large
dish. Garnish with lemon wedges.
Serve with a green salad. Serves 4.

Serving size:	1 cup
Exchanges:	1 starch/bread
	4 lean meat
Calories:	300

Quick Paella

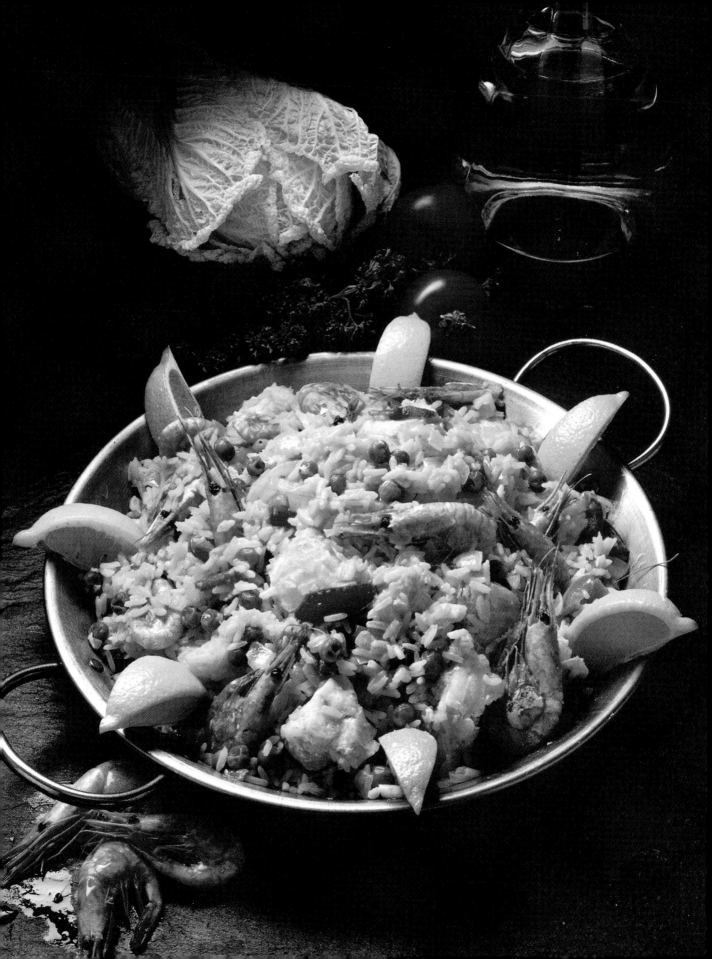

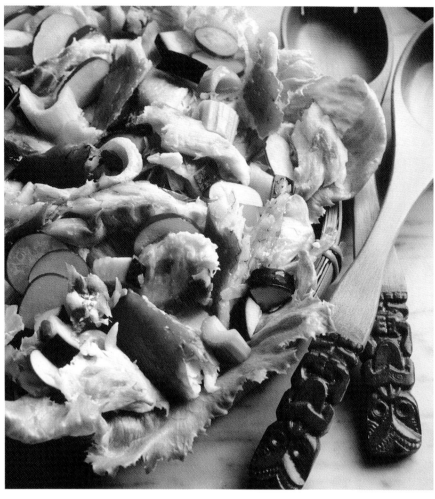

Smoked Fish Salad

FRESH SPINACH PESTO

2 cups (packed) raw spinach, rinsed and trimmed
1 garlic clove, peeled
1/2 cup chopped fresh parsley
3 teaspoons dried basil
Pinch of nutmeg
2 teaspoons low-cal Italian salad dressing
2 cups hot cooked high-protein linguini or spaghetti
2 tablespoons grated Parmesan cheese
2 cups pot cheese (uncreamed cottage cheese)
Salt and freshly ground black pepper
4 teaspoons dry-roasted sunflower seeds

1. Combine spinach, garlic, parsley, basil, nutmeg, and salad dressing in blender or food processor (using the steel blade). Cover and process until finely minced.

2. Return hot, drained, cooked pasta, unrinsed, to the pot it was cooked in. Stir in Parmesan cheese until well coated. Stir in pot cheese. And chopped spinach mixture (seasoned to taste). Stir over very low heat until warmed through.

3. Spoon onto a plate and serve immediately. Sprinkle with sunflower seeds. Serves 2.

Serving size:	1 cup	
Exchanges:	2 starch/bread	
	2 medium-fat meat	
	1/2 fruit	
Calories:	340	

SMOKED FISH SALAD

2 pounds smoked fish
1 large unpeeled cucumber, diced
12 radishes, sliced thinly
1 bunch celery, cut into 1/2-inch pieces
6 spring onions, sliced thinly
1/2 pint mayonnaise
Lettuce leaves

1. Place the fish in a large saucepan, add sufficient water to cover. Bring to a boil, cover, and simmer over low heat for 10 to 15 minutes, or until the fish flakes easily. Cool, then flake coarsely.

2. Mix the fish and vegetables together in a large bowl. Gently mix in the mayonnaise.

3. Line a serving dish with lettuce leaves and pile the salad on top. Serve chilled. Serves 10 to 12.

Serving size:	3 ounces
Exchanges:	3 medium-fat meat
	1 fat
Calories:	270

SURPRISE POCKETS

4 round crispy rolls
4 tablespoons butter or margarine
4 eggs
1 tablespoon milk
Salt and freshly ground black pepper
2 tomatoes, skinned and chopped
1 tablespoon chopped parsley

1. Preheat oven to 350 degrees.
2. Slice a small round off the top of the rolls. Scoop out some of the inside crumb. Melt 2 tablespoons butter or margarine and brush inside of rolls. Bake in a 350 degree oven for 5 minutes.

3. Melt remaining 2 tablespoons butter or margarine in saucepan. Combine eggs, milk, salt, and pepper. Add to butter or margarine. Cook gently, stirring all the time, until eggs become soft and creamy. Stir in tomatoes and parsley.
4. Pile egg mixture into the hot rolls, replace the lids, and serve hot. Serves 4.

Serving size:	1 serving
Exchanges:	2 starch/bread
	1 medium-fat meat
	1 vegetable
	3 fat
Calories:	395

Surprise Pockets

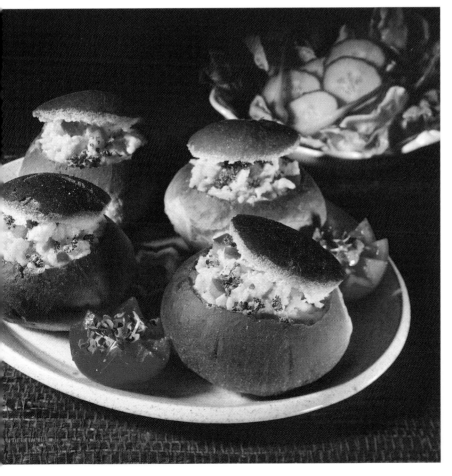

APPLE-GLAZED MINTED ROAST LEG OF LAMB

1 garlic clove, minced (optional)
4- to 7-pound leg of lamb (lean only)
6-ounce can apple juice concentrate, defrosted, undiluted
1 tablespoon dried mint flakes
Salt and freshly ground black pepper

1. Preheat oven to 325 degrees.
2. If desired, garlic can be cut into slivers and inserted in the meat with a pointed sharp knife before roasting. Leave on the paper-like skin covering the leg of lamb. This covering retains moisture. Place the lamb on a rack in a roasting pan. Insert a thermometer in the thickest part, not touching the bone. Roast, uncovered, with no water added, for about 30 minutes per pound. After $1^{1}/_{2}$ to 2 hours, drain fat from pan.
3. Combine remaining ingredients and pour over the lamb. Continue to bake, basting often, until meat thermometer registers 140 degrees for rare or 160 for medium. Lamb is best served with some pinkness remaining.
4. Remove to a cutting board and wait 15 minutes before carving. Skim fat from pan juices and discard. Serve juices as a sauce. Serves 12.

Serving size:	3 ounces
Exchanges:	3 medium-fat meat
Calories:	225

EGGPLANT PARMESAN

1 small eggplant, unpeeled, cut into
¹/2-inch slices
³/4 cup tomato sauce
1 small onion, peeled and sliced
1 small bell pepper, seeded and sliced
4-ounce can mushrooms, drained
Garlic salt and black pepper to taste
Pinch of basil and oregano
3 ounces shredded mozzarella cheese,
part-skim
1 tablespoon grated Parmesan cheese

1. Preheat oven to 400 degrees.

2. Bake eggplant slices in single layer on a nonstick baking sheet, uncovered, 15 to 20 minutes, until soft.

3. Meanwhile, combine tomato sauce, onion, bell pepper, mushrooms, and seasonings in a saucepan. Simmer 15 minutes.

4. Place half of the eggplant slices in a layer on the bottom of a nonstick casserole dish sprayed with cooking spray. Pour half the tomato sauce mixture over eggplant, and sprinkle with half the cheeses. Repeat these layers. Bake at 350 degrees, uncovered, for 30 minutes. Serves 4.

Serving size:	6 ounces
Exchanges:	¹/2 starch/bread
	1 lean meat
	1 vegetable
Calories:	120

SCRUMPTIOUS SIDE DISHES

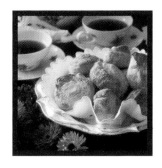

An appetizer introduces the meal, a side dish
complements it. Everyday meals often do
without one or the other, but holiday meals
allow us to savor them both.

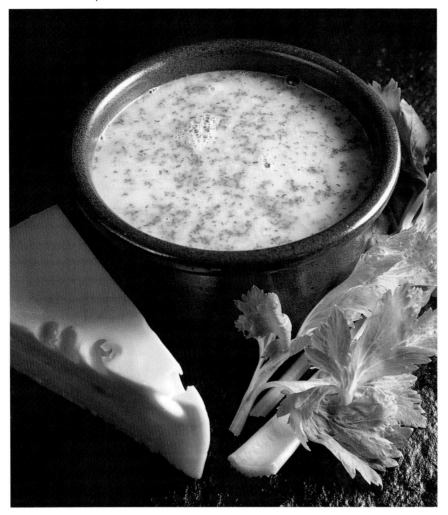

Swiss Cheese Soup

MANHATTAN CLAM CHOWDER

3 cans (7 ounces each) minced clams
3 medium potatoes, peeled and diced
3 medium carrots, peeled and diced
4 medium stalks celery, chopped
16-ounce can tomatoes
1 tablespoon bacon-flavored bits
2 teaspoons salt
¹/₂ teaspoon thyme leaves
¹/₄ teaspoon black pepper
4 cups water

1. In a large kettle or Dutch oven, combine all ingredients. Cover and simmer for 1 hour. Serves 8.

Serving size:	1 cup
Exchanges:	1 starch/bread
	1 vegetable
Calories:	105

SWISS CHEESE SOUP

1 onion, peeled and finely chopped
1 tablespoon margarine
3 tablespoons flour
4 cups vegetable or chicken stock
1¹/₄ cups grated Swiss cheese
1 egg yolk
¹/₃ cup sour cream
Shredded celery and chopped parsley for garnish

1. Saute the onion in margarine. Stir in the flour when the onion has become transparent. Cover with stock, stirring constantly. Simmer for 5 to 6 minutes.

2. Stir in the cheese and let it melt. Do not allow it to boil. Remove the pan from the heat. Stir in the egg yolk and sour cream.

3. Serve immediately, garnished with celery and parsley. Serves 4.

Serving size:	1¹/₄ cup
Exchanges:	1 starch/bread
	2 medium-fat meat
	2 fat
Calories:	320

MUSHROOMS STUFFED WITH HAM

4 large mushrooms
4 tablespoons butter or margarine
1 small onion, chopped
1 tablespoon flour
¹/₂ cup milk
Small red bell pepper
¹/₄ cup chopped cooked ham
1 tablespoon chopped parsley
Salt and freshly ground black pepper
5 tablespoons fresh bread crumbs

1. Preheat oven to 350 degrees. Grease a shallow baking dish.

2. Rinse mushrooms. Remove stems and set aside. Put mushroom caps, upside down, in baking dish.

Dot with 2 tablespoons of butter. Bake for 10 minutes.

3. Meanwhile, heat the remaining butter in a saucepan. Fry the onion until softened. Stir in the flour and cook, stirring, for 2 to 3 minutes. Blend in the milk and bring to a boil, stirring constantly. Boil for 2 minutes.

4. Chop the mushroom stalks.

Mushrooms Stuffed with Ham

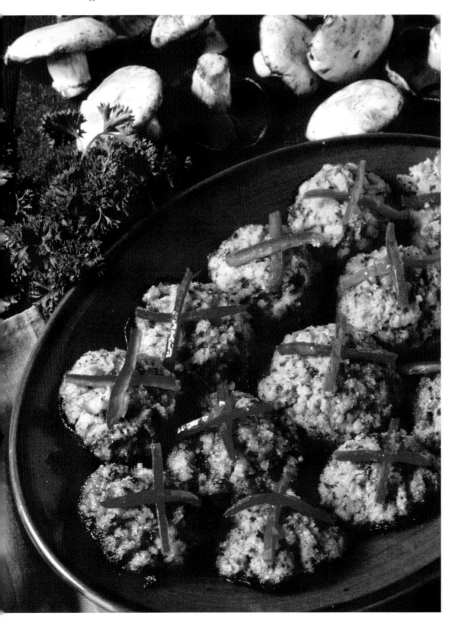

Slice red pepper in half; use one half for garnish strips. Chop the remaining red pepper. Combine pepper, mushroom stems, ham, parsley, salt, pepper and bread crumbs with the sauce. Scoop stuffing into each cap.

5. Return to oven and bake 15 to 20 minutes more. Serve hot, and garnish with pepper. Serves 4.

NOTE: Do not rinse mushrooms until ready for use.

Serving size:	¹/2 cup
Exchanges:	2 vegetable
	2 fat
Calories:	140

CLAM-STUFFED MUSHROOMS OREGANATA

1 pound large, fresh mushrooms
8-ounce can minced clams, drained
¹/8 teaspoon dried oregano
¹/8 teaspoon garlic powder,
or instant garlic
Salt and freshly ground black pepper
2 tablespoons grated Romano cheese
1 tablespoon red wine vinegar
1 slice high-fiber bread, stale or toasted,
processed, or rolled into crumbs

1. Preheat oven to 375 degrees.
2. Remove stems from mushrooms and set caps aside. Chop the stems finely. Combine chopped stems with all other ingredients and toss lightly. Stuff filling into caps.
3. Arrange mushrooms, stuffing side up, on a shallow nonstick tray. Bake for 20 to 25 minutes. Serves 3 to 4.

Serving size:	6 ounces
Exchanges:	1 starch/bread
	1 lean meat
Calories:	135

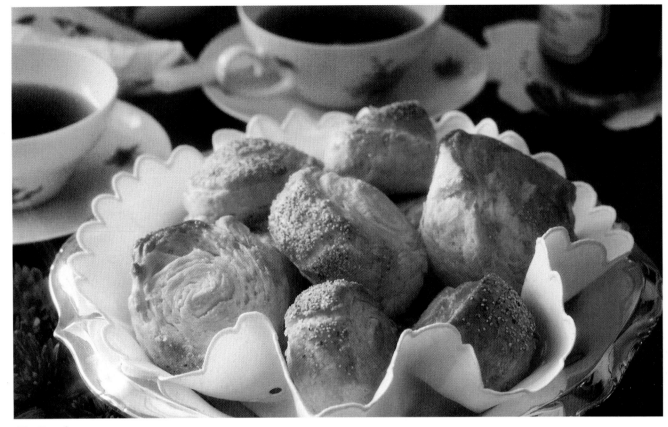

Tea Bread

MARINATED MUSHROOMS

1 pound fresh mushrooms, sliced
2 green onions, sliced
1/3 cup vegetable oil
1/3 cup white wine vinegar
2 tablespoons minced parsley
1/2 teaspoon dry mustard
1/2 teaspoon dried basil
Salt and freshly ground black pepper

1. Place all ingredients in large mixing bowl, stirring to combine. Chill several hours. Serves 8.

Serving size:	1/2 cup
Exchanges:	1 vegetable
	1 fat
Calories:	70

OYSTERS BALTIMORE

4 slices bacon
18 raw oysters
3 tablespoons chili sauce
1 tablespoon Worcestershire sauce
6 tablespoons heavy cream
1/2 teaspoon dried tarragon
2 tablespoons lemon juice
Salt and freshly ground black pepper

1. Fry sliced bacon until crisp in a medium skillet. Crumble bacon for use as a garnish. Pour off all but 2 tablespoons fat from skillet.

2. Add oysters and their juice to skillet. Cook over medium heat until almost all the juice is gone.

3. Add the remaining ingredients to the oysters and simmer for 5 minutes until flavors have blended.

Season to taste. Garnish with bacon and serve. Serves 4 to 6.

Serving size:	3
Exchanges:	1 vegetable
	1 fat
Calories:	70

CRANBERRY HOLIDAY SALAD

2 cups raw cranberries
1 orange, peeled and thinly sliced
1 cup water
3/4 cup sugar
1 envelope unflavored gelatin
1/4 cup cold water
1/2 cup sliced seedless grapes
1 cup diced celery
1/4 cup chopped nuts

1. Combine cranberries, orange slices, and water in covered saucepan. Cook until cranberry skins pop open. Press through fine sieve. Return liquid to saucepan, add sugar and bring to boil.

2. Soften gelatin in cold water in large mixing bowl. Add hot cranberries, and stir until gelatin is dissolved. Chill until syrupy.

2. Add remaining ingredients and turn into a ring mold. Chill until firm. Unmold and garnish as desired. Serves 6.

Serving size:	3 ounces
Exchanges:	1 vegetable
	2 fruit
Calories:	145

GINGERED PEAR RING

2 envelopes unflavored gelatin
Water
3¹/₂ cups canned pineapple juice
¹/₂ cup sugar
1 piece ginger root (about 2 inches long), peeled and sliced
¹/₄ cup fresh lemon juice
2 medium pears, unpeeled and cut into ¹/₂-inch cubes (about 2 cups)

1. Soften gelatin in ¹/₂ cup cold water. Place pineapple juice, sugar and ginger in a small saucepan. Bring to a boil. Reduce heat and simmer for 5 minutes; strain out ginger. Mix lemon juice and soften gelatin. Refrigerate until mixture begins to thicken.

2. Fold pears into gelatin mixture. Pour into a 1-quart ring mold. Chill

until firm and ready to serve. Just before serving, unmold onto a serving plate. (Diced peaches or apples may be substituted for the pears.) Serves 6.

Serving size:	3 ounces
Exchanges:	1¹/₂ fruit
Calories:	90

TEA BREAD

²/₃ cup milk
1 cake compressed yeast
1 egg
1 tablespoon sugar
¹/₂ teaspoon salt
2 cups flour
5 tablespoons butter
1 beaten egg
Poppy seeds

1. Heat the milk to lukewarm. Dissolve the yeast in the milk. Add the egg, sugar, salt, and flour and knead well. Let stand and rise in warm place for about 20 minutes.

2. Preheat the oven to 400 degrees.

3. Punch down the dough and knead again. Roll it out into a rectangle about 10 x 16 inches. Cut the butter into small pieces and lay them out over half the dough. Fold the other half over the buttered half. Roll the dough and fold it together into 3 layers. Repeat 4 or 5 more times.

4. Finally, roll out the dough so that it is about 12 x 30 inches. Fold it lengthwise into 3 layers. Cut the dough into 2-inch wide pieces and let it rise on a baking sheet for 15 minutes. Brush with an egg and sprinkle

with poppy seeds. Bake for 15 minutes. Makes 16 small buns.

Serving size:	1 bun
Exchanges:	1 starch/bread
	1 fat
Calories:	125

SWEET CREAM BISCUITS

4 cups flour
1 teaspoon salt
2 tablespoons baking powder
1¹/₂ cups heavy cream
¹/₄ cup water

1. Preheat the oven to 450 degrees.

2. Sift the flour, salt, and baking powder and place in a large mixing bowl. Stir in the cream with a fork, just until the flour is moistened. Add water, if necessary, until mixture is consistency of fine crumbs.

3. Knead on a lightly floured surface, about 10 times. Roll out ³/₄ inch thick; cut with a small floured cutter. Bake on an ungreased baking sheet for 12 minutes, or until golden brown. Remove from oven and serve immediately. Makes 36 small biscuits.

Serving size:	1 biscuit
Exchanges:	1¹/₂ fruit
	1 fat
Calories:	135

STUFFED PEARS

3 large, ripe pears, halved and cored
Juice of half a lemon
2 firm apples, cored and diced
2 to 3 stalks celery, diced
6 1/2 ounces crabmeat
1 tablespoon minced onion
1 tablespoon minced parsley
French salad dressing
12 lettuce leaves

1. Scoop out some of the flesh from each pear half. Brush halves with lemon juice.

2. Place pear flesh in a large mixing bowl. Add apples, celery, crabmeat, onion, and parsley. Add enough French dressing to moisten; mix well.

3. Spoon into pear halves, arrange on a bed of lettuce leaves and serve. Serves 6.

Serving size:	1/2 pear, 1 ounce crabmeat
Exchanges:	1 medium-fat meat
	1 fruit
Calories:	135

FRENCH BUNS

5 1/4 tablespoons margarine or butter
2 cups milk
2 cakes compressed yeast
5 2/3 to 6 cups flour
2 teaspoons salt

1. Melt butter in a pot. Add milk and allow mixture to become lukewarm.

2. Place yeast in dish. Add 2 tablespoons warm milk mixture. Then return to pot of milk. Add most of flour and salt. Work into a smooth dough and let rise in a draft-free place for about 40 minutes.

3. Knead dough on a baking table. Divide dough into 4 parts. Roll each dough piece out into a long roll and cut each roll into 8 pieces. Dip pieces in rest of flour. Place them on a greased baking sheet. Let rise for about 30 minutes.

4. Preheat oven to 425 degrees.

5. Bake for about 8 to 10 minutes. Serves 32.

Serving size:	1 bun
Exchanges:	2 starch/bread
Calories:	160

CORN BREAD, CORN, AND MUSHROOM STUFFING

2 cups crumbled corn bread
2 cups white bread crumbs
1 1/2 cups whole corn kernels
1 1/2 cups sliced fresh mushrooms
4 tablespoons butter or margarine, melted
Salt, freshly ground black pepper, and 1/4 teaspoon of cayenne pepper
2 tablespoons fresh chopped mixed thyme and sage, or 2 teaspoons dried
2 large eggs, beaten
6 to 8 tablespoons chicken stock

1. Combine corn bread, white bread crumbs, corn and mushrooms. Stir in melted butter.

2. Add salt, pepper, cayenne pepper, herbs, eggs, and enough stock to make a moist but not runny mixture. Spoon this mixture into cavity; skewer shut. Makes 1 cup.

Serving size:	1/2 cup
Exchanges:	1 starch/bread
	1 vegetable
	2 fat
Calories:	195

YORKSHIRE PUDDING

1 cup sifted flour
1 teaspoon salt
2 large eggs
1 cup milk
1/4 cup roast beef drippings

1. Preheat oven to 425 degrees.

2. Combine flour and salt in a large mixing bowl. Beat eggs and milk together and stir into dry ingredients. Beat until smooth. Spoon drippings into 8 x 10-inch baking pan.

Pour in batter. Bake for 25 to 30 minutes.

3. Alternatively, add mixture directly into pan with roast 30 minutes before the roast is ready. Cook with beef until done. Pudding should puff up and be crisp on top. Serves 4 to 6.

Serving size:	4 ounces
Exchanges:	2 starch/bread
	2 fat
Calories:	250

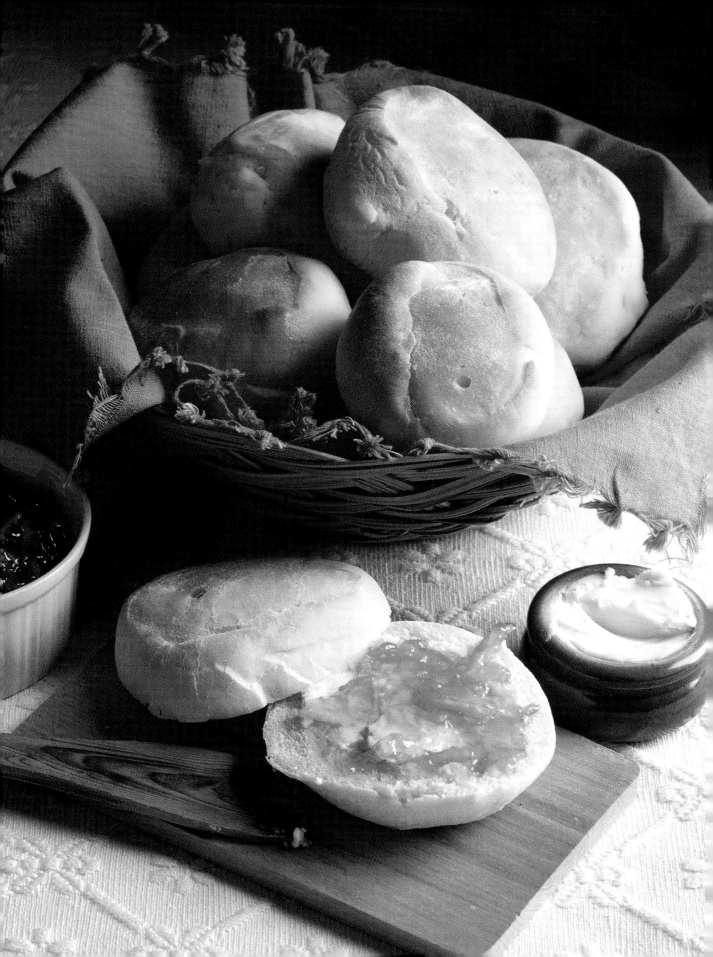

ROASTING PAN BREAD

6 cakes compressed yeast
7 tablespoons butter or margarine
4 cups lukewarm water
1 bottle (16 ounces) lukewarm beer
4 teaspoons salt
2 tablespoons light corn syrup
8 cups whole wheat flour

1. Place the yeast in a large mixing bowl. Melt the butter in a small saucepan and add the water and beer. Dissolve the yeast in 2 tablespoons of the liquid. When yeast foams, add remaining liquid, salt, and corn syrup. Stir in enough flour to form a soft dough.

2. Preheat oven to 475 degrees.

3. Place all the dough in a 12 x 16-inch greased roasting pan. Flatten and push dough into pan with a floured hand. Prick the surface with a fork. Cover dough with a damp cloth. Let rise in a warm place for about 1 hour.

4. Bake at 475 degrees for about 15 minutes, or until the bread turns golden. Lower heat to 400 degrees and bake for another 30 minutes.

5. Cool bread in pan on rack. When cold, cut it into 4 pieces. Serves 6 to 8.

Serving size:	2 ounces
Exchanges:	2 starch/bread
	1 fat
Calories:	205

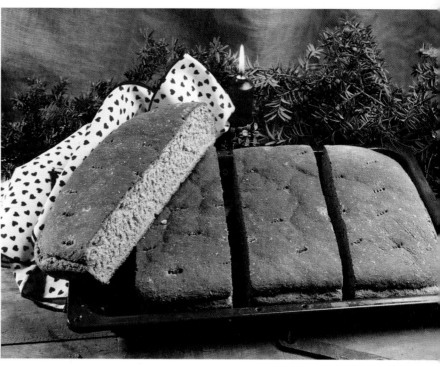

Roasting Pan Bread

APPLE STUFFING

3 cups diced bread
5 tablespoons butter or margarine
1 tablespoon lemon juice
1 teaspoon salt
1 cup chopped tart apples
1 teaspoon chopped fresh mint, or 1/2 teaspoon dried

1. Combine bread, butter, lemon juice, and moisten with a little water. Add salt, apples, and mint. Spoon loosely into cavity; skewer shut. Makes about 4 1/2 cups.

Serving size:	1/2 cup
Exchanges:	2 starch/bread
	1 fruit
	2 fat
Calories:	310

OYSTER STUFFING

1/2 cup butter or margarine
1 large onion, peeled and chopped
1/2 cup sliced celery
5 cups fresh bread crumbs
1/4 cup chopped fresh parsley
Salt and freshly ground black pepper
Juice of half a lemon
2 cups raw oysters in own liquid
White wine or chicken stock

1. Melt butter in a large skillet. Saute onion and celery until soft and golden.

2. Place bread crumbs in a large mixing bowl. Add onion and celery. Stir in parsley, salt, pepper, and lemon juice. Cut oysters in half if very large. Combine the oysters and liquid with bread crumbs. If too dry, add white wine or stock for more moisture.

3. Spoon stuffing into cavity of bird; skewer shut. For a very large turkey, double this recipe. For non-poultry meat entrees, use the basic recipe and bake in a baking dish at 350 degrees for 30 minutes. Serve immediately. Makes 8 cups.

Serving size:	1/2 cup
Exchanges:	1 starch/bread
	1 vegetable
	2 fat
Calories:	195

SAUSAGE MEAT STUFFING

1 pound fresh pork sausage meat
1 cup chopped celery
1 large onion, peeled and chopped
1/4 cup butter or margarine, melted
1 turkey or other poultry liver
2 to 3 tablespoons chopped fresh mixed parsley and thyme, or 2 teaspoons dried
2 cups bread crumbs
1 large egg, beaten
Juice of half a lemon

1. Combine sausage and celery in a large mixing bowl. Melt butter in a skillet. Saute onion and liver for 2 to 3 minutes. Remove and cool slightly.

2. Cut liver into small pieces. Combine liver and onion with sausage mixture. Add herbs, bread crumbs, egg and juice to moisten. Spoon stuffing into cavity; skewer shut. Makes 4 cups.

Serving size:	1/2 cup
Exchanges:	1/2 starch/bread
	2 medium-fat meat
	2 fat
Calories:	280

Oyster Stuffing

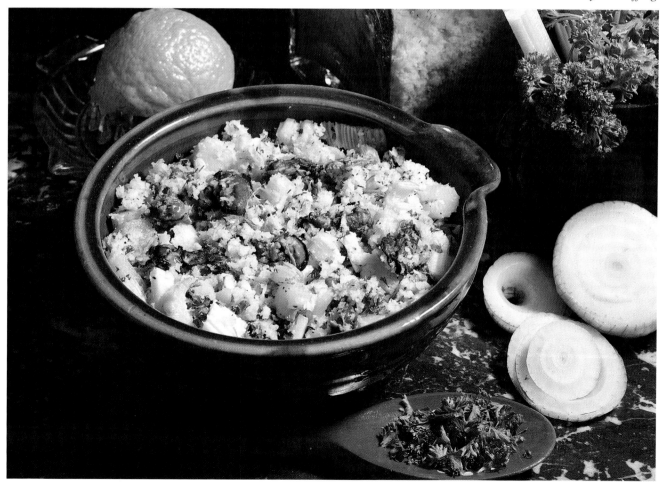

ROANOKE PECAN STUFFING

4 cups chicken stock
1 carrot, quartered
2 bay leaves
Salt to taste
1 cup wild rice
1/2 cup butter or margarine
1 large onion, chopped
4 cups sliced mushrooms
4 stalks celery, sliced
1/4 cup chopped parsley
2 teaspoons chopped fresh sage, or
1/2 teaspoon dried
4 cups cubed corn bread or corn bread stuffing mix
2 cups cubed whole wheat bread
2 cups halved or chopped pecans
Salt and freshly ground black pepper

1. Place 3 cups chicken stock in large saucepan with carrot, bay leaves, and salt. Bring to a boil and add wild rice. Cook according to package directions for about 40 minutes, or until soft. Remove the carrot and bay leaves.

2. Meanwhile, place butter in large skillet and saute onion, mushrooms, and celery until soft. Add the parsley, sage, and remaining chicken stock to the mushroom mixture and simmer 8 to 10 minutes.

3. Place corn bread, whole wheat bread, pecans, and cooked rice in a large mixing bowl. Add onion mixture. Season with salt and pepper. For moister dressing, add more chicken stock, as desired. Use as stuffing or bake in a greased 2-quart baking dish at 325 degrees for about 30 minutes. Makes about 12 cups.

Serving size:	1/2 cup
Exchanges:	1 starch/bread
	1 vegetable
	1 fat
Calories:	150

WILD RICE STUFFING

3/4 cups coarsely chopped pecans
1/4 cup butter or margarine
1 large onion, peeled and minced
1 cup finely chopped celery
1/4 pound mushrooms cut into 1/2 inch cubes (about 2 cups)
1 turkey liver, chopped (optional)
Salt and freshly ground black pepper
4 cups cooked wild rice

1. Toast the pecans in a large skillet and set pecans aside.

2. Place the butter in the skillet and add the onion and celery. Cook, stirring, until soft. Add the mushrooms and chopped liver. Season with salt and pepper; cook about 5 minutes. Add the cooked wild rice and pecans; blend thoroughly. Makes 8 cups.

Serving size:	1/2 cup
Exchanges:	1 starch/bread
	2 fat
Calories:	170

LEEKS AU GRATIN

8 to 12 leeks, rinsed and trimmed
3 tablespoons butter or margarine
2 tablespoons flour
1 cup milk
1 cup grated Cheddar cheese
Salt and freshly ground black pepper
1/2 to 1 teaspoon Dijon mustard
Juice of half a lemon
1/4 cup bread crumbs

1. Preheat oven to 375 degrees. Grease a 2-quart baking dish.

2. Trim tops off leeks. Place leeks in a large saucepan. Boil in salted water to cover until tender. Drain well and place in baking dish.

3. Make the sauce: Place 2 tablespoons of butter in a small saucepan and melt. Add the flour and milk. Stir until smooth and well blended. Add cheese, salt, pepper, mustard and lemon juice.

4. Pour sauce over the leeks. Dot remaining butter on top. Sprinkle with bread crumbs and bake about 25 minutes until top is crisp and brown. Serves 4 to 6.

Serving size:	6 ounces
Exchanges:	1 starch/bread
	2 medium-fat meat
	3 fat
Calories:	365

LEEKS WITH MUSTARD GREENS AND CRESS

1 pound small leeks
Water
Salt
Mustard greens and watercress

DRESSING
1 tablespoon vinegar
1/2 teaspoon salt
1/2 teaspoon tarragon
1 tablespoon water

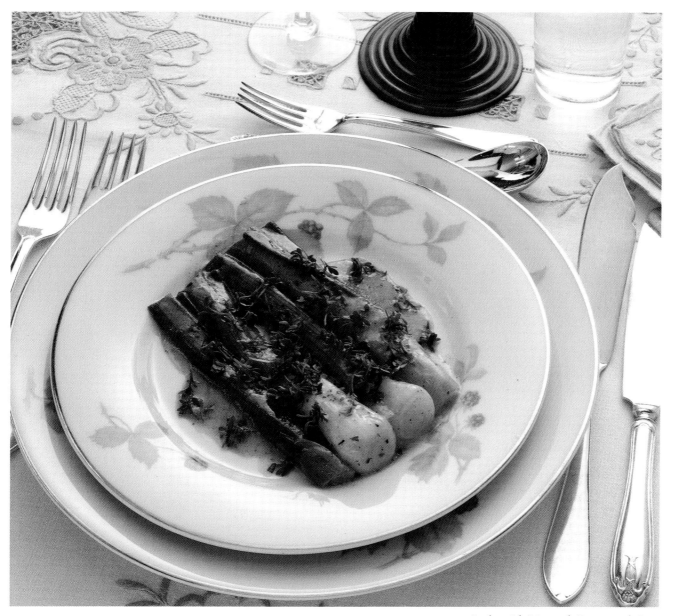

Leeks with Mustard Greens and Cress

1 teaspoon mustard
3 to 4 tablespoons oil

1. Wash leeks well. Trim root ends and most of the green. In a wide, shallow pan, bring water to a boil. Add 2 teaspoons salt per quart of water. Divide leeks into 2 or 3 pieces, if they are too long to fit in pan.

Cook for about 2 minutes, until tender. Do not overcook.

2. Blend ingredients for the dressing and beat for a few minutes to allow salt to dissolve. Drain leeks and place in a dish.

3. Pour dressing over leeks while they are still hot. Allow them to get cold and marinate for an hour or

two. Cut some mustard greens and watercress onto the leeks when serving and offer with bread and butter. Serves 4.

Serving size:	½ cup
Exchanges:	½ starch/bread
Calories:	40

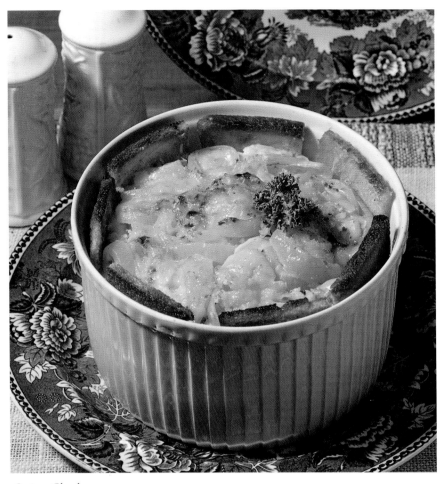

Onion Charlotte

ONION CHARLOTTE

4 large Bermuda onions, peeled and sliced thick
1 cup plus 1 tablespoon milk
$1/4$ cup water
2 tablespoons cornstarch
3 tablespoons butter or margarine
Salt and freshly ground black pepper
$1/8$ teaspoon grated nutmeg
$1/8$ teaspoon ground cinnamon
$1/4$ cup vegetable oil
4 to 5 slices stale white bread, crusts removed
3 tablespoons grated Parmesan cheese
2 tablespoons bread crumbs

1. Preheat oven to 400 degrees.
2. Place the onions in a large saucepan. Add enough water to cover and bring to a boil. Cook for 2 to 3 minutes. Drain off water and return onions to pan. Add 1 cup milk and $1/4$ cup water, cover, and simmer for 10 to 15 minutes, or until onions are tender.
3. Mix remaining milk with cornstarch and stir until mixture becomes a smooth paste. Add to onions and stir. Bring to a boil. Add 2 tablespoons butter, salt, pepper, nutmeg, and cinnamon.
4. Pour oil into a small skillet. Fry bread until brown on both sides. Arrange the bread in the bottom and around the sides of a greased 2-quart baking dish. Pour in onion mixture.
5. Mix cheese and bread crumbs together in a small mixing bowl. Then sprinkle over top of onion mixture. Melt remaining butter and drizzle over top.

GREEN PEAS WITH LETTUCE

1 tablespoon vegetable oil
$1/4$ pound Canadian bacon, cut into 1-inch cubes
3 cups fresh or frozen green peas
6 small white pearl onions, peeled
head of loose leaf lettuce
$1/2$ cup water
$1/2$ teaspoon salt
$1/4$ teaspoon freshly ground black pepper
$1/2$ teaspoon sugar
1 tablespoon finely chopped fresh parsley

1. Heat oil in medium skillet. Add bacon pieces, and saute until lightly browned. Add peas, onions, tender inner lettuce leaves, water, salt, pepper, and sugar. Cover; cook for 10 minutes or until peas are tender.
2. Drain peas and put into serving dish. Sprinkle with parsley. Serves 6.

Serving size:	$1/2$ cup
Exchanges:	1 starch/bread
	$1/2$ medium-fat meat
Calories:	118

6. Bake for 35 to 40 minutes or until top is crusty and brown. Serves 4.

Serving size:	6 ounces
Exchanges:	1 starch/bread
	2 vegetable
	3 fat
Calories:	265

PUFFED CAULIFLOWER CHEESE

Medium head of cauliflower, washed, trimmed, and quartered
1/4 cup butter or margarine
2 tablespoons flour
1 cup milk
Salt and freshly ground black pepper
1/4 cup white bread crumbs
3 large eggs, separated
1 cup grated Swiss cheese

1. Preheat oven to 400 degrees. Grease a 2-quart baking dish.
2. Divide cauliflower quarters into florets. Boil in salted water to cover until tender. Drain.
3. Melt the butter in a large saucepan. Add the flour, and stir over low heat for 2 minutes. Remove from heat, add milk gradually, and stir until smooth. Return to the heat, and cook until boiling, stirring constantly. Add salt and pepper to taste and most of the bread crumbs.
4. Stir in the egg yolks, cheese, and cauliflower. Place egg whites in a large mixing bowl and beat until stiff. Fold into mixture. Spoon into baking dish and sprinkle with remaining bread crumbs.

5. Bake for about 30 minutes or until puffy and brown. Serves 4.

Serving size:	1 cup
Exchanges:	1 starch/bread
	2 medium-fat meat
	2 fat
Calories:	320

JANSSON'S TEMPTATION

3 tablespoons butter or margarine
2 medium onions, peeled and sliced very thin
4 or 5 large baking potatoes, peeled and grated
15 to 18 anchovy fillets
1 cup heavy cream
Freshly ground white pepper

1. Preheat oven to 300 degrees. Grease a 9-inch pie tin.
2. Place 2 tablespoons butter in a large skillet. Saute onions until golden. Arrange thin layers of grated potatoes, onions, anchovies, and then top with potatoes. Dot with remaining butter and sprinkle with pepper.
3. Bake for 50 minutes. After first 10 minutes pour in half the cream; after second 10 minutes, pour in remaining cream. Serves 4.

Serving size:	1/2 cup
Exchanges:	1 starch/bread
	1/2 vegetable
	3 fat
Calories:	228

Puffed Cauliflower Cheese

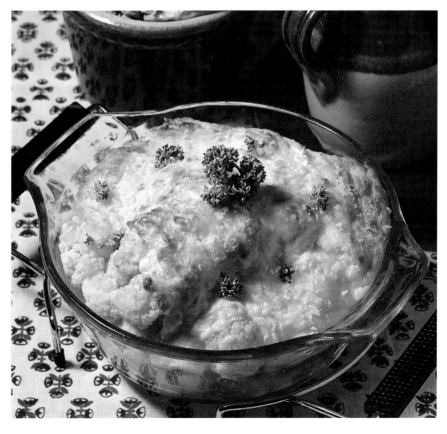

BROCCOLI-POTATO CASSEROLE

1 10-ounce package frozen chopped broccoli
¼ cup butter or margarine
1 small onion, peeled and chopped
1½ cups mashed potatoes
Salt and freshly ground black pepper

1. Cook the broccoli according to package directions; drain. Melt butter in small skillet and saute onion until golden.

2. Combine potatoes, broccoli, onion, salt, and pepper in top of double boiler. Cover and reheat over boiling water. Serves 4.

Serving size:	½ cup
Exchanges:	½ starch/bread
	3 fat
Calories:	175

HOLIDAY RICE

3 cups uncooked long-grain white rice
6 cups boiling water
1 pound country sausage links
1 cup chopped celery
2 medium onions, peeled and chopped
1 green bell pepper, diced
1 large egg, beaten
Salt and freshly ground black pepper

1. Add rice to boiling water in large saucepan. Lower heat, cover. Simmer until rice is tender, about 20 minutes. Drain rice in colander.

2. Fry sausages in a large skillet. Remove sausages and drain on paper towels. Pour off some of the fat.

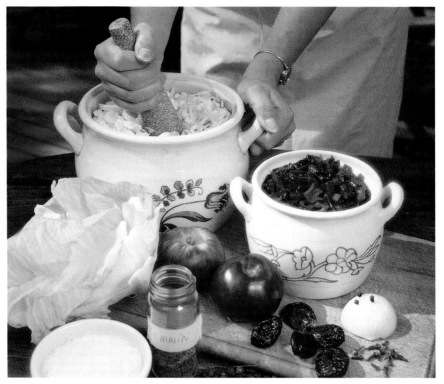

Sauerkraut

Saute celery, onions, and pepper in remaining fat until lightly browned. Add the rice, stirring well for about 3 minutes. Remove to a serving bowl.

3. Add the egg, salt and pepper to the skillet. Mix well and cook until firm. Stir into the rice mixture and serve immediately.

4. If desired, make this dish ahead, and place rice-sausage-egg mixture into a greased baking dish, cover with foil, and freeze. Reheat in oven and serve. Serves 10 to 12.

Serving size:	5 ounces
Exchanges:	1 starch/bread
	1 medium-fat meat
	2 fat
Calories:	245

EPICUREAN WILD RICE

⅓ cup butter or margarine
½ cup minced fresh parsley
½ cup chopped scallions
1 cup diagonally sliced celery
1¼ cups wild rice
1½ cups chicken stock
1½ cups boiling water
1 teaspoon salt
½ teaspoon dried marjoram
½ cup dry sherry

1. Preheat oven to 350 degrees.

2. Melt the butter in a large saucepan. Add the parsley, scallions, and celery. Saute until soft but not brown. Spoon into a greased 3-quart baking dish. Add the rice, stock, water, salt, and marjoram and cover tightly with foil.

3. Bake about 45 minutes, or until rice is tender. Stir occasionally and add boiling water if necessary.

4. Remove foil. Stir in sherry. Bake for 5 minutes. Serves 6.

Serving size:	1/2 cup
Exchanges:	1 starch/bread
	1 fat
Calories:	125

SAUERKRAUT

CABBAGE
Several large cabbage leaves
6 1/2 to 7 pounds cabbage, rinsed, cored, and shredded
2 large tart apples, cored and sliced
3 tablespoons coarse salt
2 teaspoons caraway seeds
10 dried juniper berries

SAUERKRAUT
4 cups sauerkraut
2 cups beef broth or pork drippings
1 large onion with 1 clove inserted in it
1 teaspoon caraway seeds

1. Make sauerkraut: Layer shredded cabbage with salt, apples, caraway seeds, and juniper berries. Pound each layer hard so that the cabbage becomes juicy. Cover with the whole cabbage leaves. Place a plate on the mixture weighted with a heavy object. Let cabbage stand for 3 to 4 days at room temperature in cool place and then refrigerate. Keep cabbage at temperatures below 40 degrees to help with the pickling process.

2. After about 2 weeks, the cab-

bage has become sauerkraut and is ready to be cooked.

3. To cook sauerkraut: Rinse and drain. Place it in the broth with the onion and caraway seeds. Let simmer until soft, 30 to 45 minutes. Season as desired. Serves 4.

Serving size:	1/2 cup
Exchanges:	1/2 medium-fat meat
	2 vegetable
Calories:	88

SWEET POTATOES, APPLES, AND SAUSAGE

4 cups unpeeled, thinly sliced tart apples
4 cups unpeeled, thinly sliced sweet potatoes
2 teaspoons minced onion
2 teaspoons salt
1/2 cup maple syrup
1/2 cup apple juice
1/4 cup butter or margarine, melted
1 pound bulk pork sausage
1/3 cup dried bread crumbs

1. Preheat oven to 350 degrees.
2. Place layer of apples, then layer of sweet potatoes in a greased 2-quart baking dish. Sprinkle each layer with onion and salt. Combine the maple syrup, apple juice, and butter in a mixing bowl. Pour over apple mixture. Cover with foil and bake for 1 hour.
3. Meanwhile, crumble sausage into a large skillet and fry until brown. Drain off fat and combine sausage with bread crumbs in a mixing bowl. When the potatoes are cooked, uncover dish and spread

with the sausage. Bake uncovered another 20 minutes. Serves 6.

Serving size:	1/2 cup
Exchanges:	1 starch/bread
	1 medium-fat meat
	4 fat
Calories:	335

SWEET POTATO BALLS

Salt and freshly ground black pepper
1 teaspoon grated lemon rind
2 cups mashed sweet potatoes
8 marshmallows
1 cup bread or cracker crumbs
1 large egg, beaten
2 tablespoons water
Vegetable oil for frying

1. Combine salt and pepper with lemon rind and sweet potatoes in a large mixing bowl. Roll mixture into 8 equal-sized balls. Put 1 marshmallow into the center of each ball. Place crumbs in a large mixing bowl; roll balls in crumbs.

2. Combine the egg and water in a small mixing bowl. Dip the balls into this and roll again in crumbs. Pour 2 inches of vegetable oil into a large skillet and heat. Fry balls for about 4 minutes, or until brown and crispy. Drain on paper towels. Serves 4 to 6.

Serving size:	3 ounces
Exchanges:	1 starch/bread
	1 fruit
Calories:	140

ROASTED CHESTNUTS

*2 pounds of
fresh chestnuts*

1. Make diagonal slits on the flat side of each chestnut with a sharp paring knife.

2. Put 5 to 6 chestnuts on a foil square and wrap into a neat package. Put directly on hot coals at the edge of an open fire or in a 425-degree oven. Roast for 15 to 20 minutes. Serves 8 to 10.

Serving size:	1 ounce no shells
Exchanges:	1 medium-fat meat
	1 vegetable
	2 fat
Calories:	190

CORN CASSEROLE WITH HAM AND CHEESE

*Kernels from 6 ears of corn
3 to 4 thick slices of ham, cubed
3 large eggs
1¹/₄ cups milk
2 cups grated sharp Cheddar cheese
¹/₈ teaspoon nutmeg*

1. Preheat oven to 400 degrees.

2. Place the corn and ham in a greased 1-quart baking dish.

3. Combine the eggs and milk in a medium mixing bowl and beat. Add cheese and nutmeg. Pour this over the corn and ham. Bake for 25 minutes. Serves 3 to 4.

Serving size:	1 cup
Exchanges:	1 starch/bread
	3 medium-fat meat
	2 fat
Calories:	395

Corn Casserole with Ham and Cheese

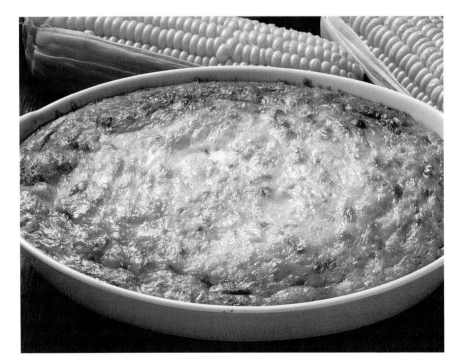

OVEN-ROASTED ROOT VEGETABLES

*1 pound carrots,
trimmed, washed, and scraped
1 pound beets,
trimmed, washed, and peeled
²/₃ pound parsnips,
trimmed and washed
¹/₄ pound celery stalks
3 tablespoons extra-virgin olive oil
¹/₂ teaspoon salt*

1. Preheat oven to 425 degrees.

2. Cut vegetables into ¹/₄-inch-wide strips.

3. Place the vegetables into a 2-quart baking dish. Pour oil over them and sprinkle with salt.

4. Bake for 25 to 30 minutes until done as desired, turning vegetables often. Sprinkle with grated Parmesan cheese. Serves 4.

Serving size:	¹/₂ cup
Exchanges:	¹/₂ starch/bread
	¹/₂ fat
Calories:	62

GOLDEN TURNIP PUDDING

*1¹/₂ pounds yellow turnips, peeled and
sliced
Boiling water to cover
2 teaspoons salt
3 eggs separated
3 tablespoons butter or margarine,
melted
1 cup dried bread crumbs
¹/₄ cup 2% milk
¹/₂ cup grated sharp Cheddar cheese*

1. Preheat oven to 350 degrees.

2. Place turnips in large saucepan and cover with boiling water. Add 1 teaspoon salt and cover. Simmer about 20 minutes, until tender. Drain and mash.

3. Place egg yolks in a large mixing bowl and beat well. Add butter, 1 teaspoon salt, bread crumbs, milk, and cheese. Stir in turnips and mix well.

4. In a small mixing bowl, beat egg whites until stiff. Fold into the turnip mixture. Scoop into a 2-quart baking dish. Place dish in a large roasting pan containing hot water. Bake for 1 hour, or until firm in center. Serves 4 to 6.

Serving size:	½ cup
Exchanges:	1½ vegetable
	2 fat
Calories:	135

BROCCOLI FRITTERS

½ cup butter or margarine
1 cup water
Salt and freshly ground black pepper
⅛ teaspoon garlic powder
1 cup flour, sifted
4 large eggs
2 packages frozen chopped broccoli
(10 ounces each), cooked according to
package directions
Vegetable oil for frying
½ cup freshly grated Parmesan cheese

1. Combine butter, water, salt and pepper to taste, and garlic powder in a large saucepan. Heat until water is boiling and butter melts. Add flour all at once and remove from heat. Stir mixture quickly until dough comes away from side of pan and forms a mound. Add eggs one at a time, beating well after each addition until mixture is smooth. Stir broccoli into dough. Chill 2 hours or overnight.

2. Pour oil into deep skillet or large saucepan to depth of 3 inches. Heat to 375 degrees. Scoop up one teaspoon of dough. Carefully drop into oil using a second spoon to place fritter. Fry one or two at a time. Fry on one side about 2 minutes; turn and fry on other. Remove with slotted spoon and drain on paper towels. Sprinkle with Parmesan cheese before serving. Serves 8.

NOTE: To use fresh broccoli, purchase two bunches and trim heads into bite-sized florets. Reserve stalks for making soup.

Serving size:	½ cup
Exchanges:	2 starch/bread
	2 fat
Calories:	250

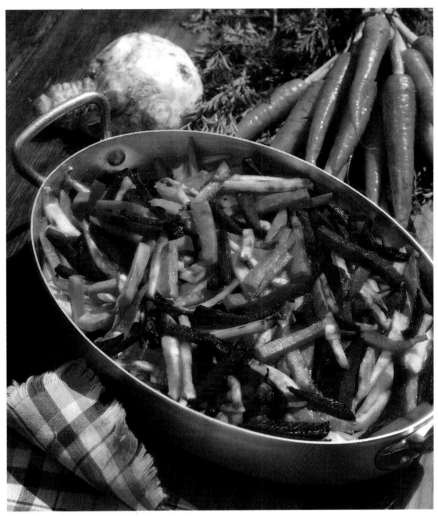

Oven Roasted Root Vegetables

SOUTHERN SWEET POTATO AND ORANGE CASSEROLE

2 cans sweet potatoes (16 ounces each), drained
1/3 cup brown sugar, firmly packed
1/4 cup butter or margarine, melted
1/2 teaspoon salt
2 tablespoons dark rum
11-ounce can mandarin oranges, drained
1/4 cup chopped pecans

1. Preheat oven to 375 degrees.
2. Place sweet potatoes in large mixing bowl and mash. Stir in 1/4 cup brown sugar, 2 tablespoons butter, salt, and rum. Stir in oranges and scoop mixture into greased 2-quart baking dish.
3. Combine pecans and remaining brown sugar and butter. Sprinkle over top. Bake for 30 minutes. Serves 8.

Serving size:	1/2 cup
Exchanges:	2 fruit
	1 fat
Calories:	165

MAPLE BUTTER SQUASH

2 large acorn squash
Extra-virgin olive oil
1/4 cup butter or margarine
1/4 cup maple syrup
Salt and freshly ground black pepper

1. Preheat oven to 350 degrees.
2. Rub the skins of each squash with olive oil to crisp skin. Place squash on a cookie sheet. Bake for 60 to 75 minutes or until tender.
3. Remove from oven. Cut in half, taking care to keep skin intact. Scoop out the seeds and fibers. Remove the flesh and mash with a fork. Blend in the butter, maple syrup, salt, and pepper.
4. Spoon equal amounts of mixture into each squash shell. Return to oven to reheat for about 5 minutes. Serves 4.

Serving size:	3/4 cup
Exchanges:	1 starch/bread
	2 fat
Calories:	170

Vegetable Fritters

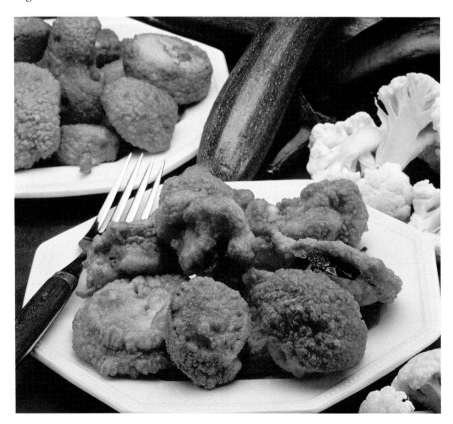

VEGETABLE FRITTERS

1 small eggplant
Salt
1 large zucchini
1/2 head cauliflower
1/2 cup flour
2 eggs
1/4 cup milk
Vegetable oil for frying

1. Slice the eggplant into thin circles. Place circles in a colander; sprinkle with salt. Set aside. Slice the zucchini and divide the cauliflower into florets.
2. Sift the flour into a large mixing bowl and add a pinch of salt. Make a well in the center. Add the eggs and mix into the flour. Gradually add milk, beating well

pie with the pastry. Make a slit in the top and decorate, if desired.

4. Bake at 425 degrees for 30 minutes. Then reduce heat to 375 degrees and bake for 1 hour. Serves 4.

Serving size:	$^1/8$ pie
Exchanges:	2 starch/bread
	2 fat
Calories:	250

SPICED BEETS

4$^1/2$ pounds beets, rinsed
Water to cover
1 piece horseradish root
Pickle juice
1$^2/3$ cups apple cider vinegar
2$^1/3$ cups water
$^1/2$ tablespoon salt
1$^1/4$ cups sugar
10 white peppercorns
8 whole cloves
5 allspice corns

1. Boil whole beets in water until almost soft. Rinse beets in cold running water and pull off skins.

2. Prepare the pickle juice by boiling together the vinegar, water, salt, sugar, and spices. Place the beets in the juice and boil them until soft. Place the beets and juice in glass jars. Put small pieces of horseradish on top. Seal jars tightly and store in cool place. Serves 8 to 10.

Serving size:	$^1/2$ cup
Exchanges:	1 fruit
Calories:	60

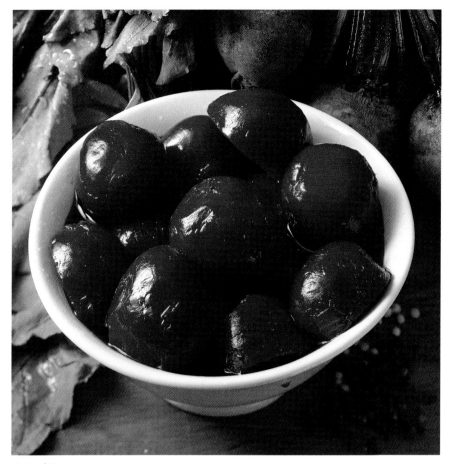

Spiced Beets

until the batter is smooth. Rinse and drain eggplant and pat dry.

3. Pour 2 inches of oil into a large skillet and heat. Dip vegetables into batter and fry pieces individually until golden. Drain on paper towels and serve immediately. Serves 4 to 6.

NOTE: For a dash of zest, offer family or guests some hot pepper sauce to sprinkle on the fritters.

Serving size:	$^1/2$ cup
Exchanges:	1 starch/bread
	$^1/2$ fat
Calories:	102

FIDGET PIE

1 pound potatoes, peeled and sliced
1 pound cooking apples, peeled, cored, and sliced
2 to 3 large onions, peeled and sliced
$^1/4$ pound bacon or ham, diced
Salt and freshly ground black pepper
1 cup beef consomme
9-inch unbaked pie shell

1. Preheat oven to 425 degrees.
2. Arrange the potatoes, apples, onions, and bacon or ham in layers in a deep 9-inch square baking dish. Season each layer with salt and pepper.
3. Add the consomme and cover

GREEN BEANS A LA GRECQUE

2 ripe tomatoes, peeled and diced
1 onion, peeled and minced
Salt (or garlic salt) and freshly ground
black pepper
¹/4 cup water
1 tablespoon minced fresh mint or
1 teaspoon dried mint
³/4 pound fresh green beans, tipped and
sliced

1. Combine all the ingredients, except beans. Cover and simmer 10 minutes.
2. Stir in beans. Simmer, uncovered, stirring often until green beans are just tender and the liquid is reduced. Serves 4.

Serving size	³/4 cup
Exchanges:	2 vegetable
Calories:	50

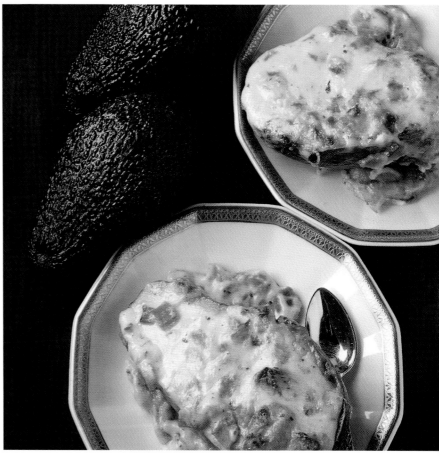

Stuffed Avocados au Gratin

STUFFED AVOCADOS AU GRATIN

4 large ripe avocados
1 package instant Hollandaise mix
4 to 6 ham slices, slivered
1 cup grated Swiss cheese

1. Preheat oven to 450 degrees.
2. Place each avocado on cutting board. With sharp paring knife, carefully slice off top third of avocado. Lift off top portion and remove; discard seeds. Scoop out avocado from tops and bottoms. Reserve bottoms. Place avocado in large mixing bowl, and cut into chunks.

3. Make Hollandaise sauce according to package directions. Put sauce in mixing bowl with avocados. Add ham. Divide the mixture evenly among the avocado bottoms. Place them on a cookie sheet, and sprinkle each generously with cheese.
4. Bake for 15 minutes. Serves 4.

Serving size:	1
Exchanges:	2 starch/bread
	3 medium-fat meat
	6 fat
Calories:	655

SPICED YELLOW SQUASH

2 packages frozen yellow squash
Artificial sweetener
Pinch of salt
¹/2 teaspoon cinnamon
¹/2 teaspoon ginger
1 tablespoon margarine

1. Defrost squash and drain off liquid. Heat in pan on top of stove and stir constantly. When heated thoroughly remove from heat.
2. Add artificial sweetener to taste, and salt, cinnamon, ginger and the margarine. Serves 8.

Serving size:	¹/₂ cup
Exchanges:	1 vegetable
Calories:	25

GRATIN VEGETABLES AND NOODLES

5 tomatoes
2 tablespoons margarine
2 onions, peeled and sliced
2 green bell peppers, diced
1 pound eggplant or squash, sliced
2 garlic cloves, crushed
2 to 3 tablespoons chili sauce
1 teaspoon salt
1 to 2 teaspoons thyme or oregano
8 ounces noodles
1 cup coarsely grated cheese

1. Dip the tomatoes in hot water. Peel off the skins. Cut the tomatoes into pieces.

2. Heat the margarine in a large pot. Saute the onions until golden yellow. Add the vegetables. Stir, and season with garlic, chili sauce, salt, and thyme or oregano. Cover and simmer over low heat for 10 to 15 minutes. Uncover and simmer 15 minutes, until the mixture thickens. If too thick, thin with water.

3. Preheat oven to 425 degrees.

4. Boil the noodles according to the package directions.

5. Grease a baking dish. Place half of the noodles in the bottom of the dish. Cover with the vegetable mixture. Top with remaining noodles and grated cheese. Bake for about 10 minutes. This dish is ideal for freezing. Serves 4 to 6.

Serving size:	1 cup
Exchanges:	2 starch/bread
	1 medium-fat meat
Calories:	235

MARINATED VEGETABLES ITALIANO

3 medium potatoes (about 1 pound)
1 cup tomato wedges
2 cups broccoli florets
1 cup mushroom slices
¹/₂ pound asparagus spears, cooked and drained
8-ounce bottle low-calorie Italian dressing
Lettuce
Celery leaves for garnish

1. Cook, peel, and slice potatoes. Combine with tomatoes, broccoli, mushrooms, and asparagus. Pour dressing over vegetables. Cover; marinate in refrigerator overnight. Drain, reserving marinade.

2. Arrange vegetables on lettuce-covered platter. Serve with reserved marinade. Garnish with celery leaves. Serves 8.

Serving size:	1 cup
Exchanges:	2 starch/bread
	1 vegetable
	1 fat
Calories:	230

Gratin Vegetables and Noodles

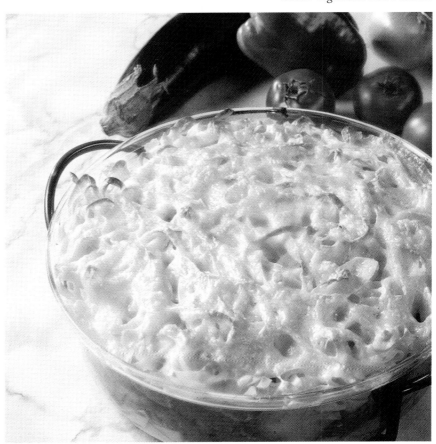

YANKEE SPOON BREAD

10-ounce package frozen corn kernels
3 cups milk
1 cup cornmeal
3 tablespoons butter or margarine
1 teaspoon baking powder
3 large eggs, separated
Salt

1. Preheat oven to 325 degrees. Grease a 1-quart baking dish.
2. Cook the corn according to package directions. Drain and cool.
3. Heat 2 cups of the milk in a saucepan. Mix the cornmeal with the remaining milk. Stir into the hot milk. Cook over medium heat until mixture thickens; stir constantly. Add butter and salt, and let cool.
4. Add corn, baking powder and slightly beaten egg yolks to cornmeal.
5. Beat the egg whites until stiff. Fold into cornmeal mixture. Pour into greased casserole dish.
6. Bake for 45 minutes. Serve immediately. Serves 6 to 8.

Serving size:	4 ounces
Exchanges:	2 starch/bread
	1 fat
Calories:	205

COUNTRY CABBAGE NOODLES

1 head green cabbage, rinsed, cored, and quartered
2 large onions, peeled and diced
1/2 cup butter or margarine
Salt and freshly ground black pepper
1/2 pound wide egg noodles

1. Cover cabbage quarters in cold, salted water. Soak for 5 minutes. Drain and grate coarsely. Cover and set aside for 30 minutes.
2. Saute the onions in a large skillet in 2 tablespoons butter until golden. Press remaining water from cabbage. Add cabbage, salt and pepper to onions. Cook, uncovered, adding butter as needed, for about 1 hour or until browned. Stir occasionally to avoid sticking.
3. Meanwhile, prepare noodles according to package directions and drain. Mix with cabbage and serve immediately. Serves 4.

Serving size:	5 ounces
Exchanges:	1 starch/bread
	2 fat
Calories:	170

HOT BRUSSELS SPROUTS IN DILLED "HOLLANDAISE" SAUCE

10 ounces fresh or defrosted brussels sprouts
Onion salt and freshly ground black pepper, to taste
1/2 cup water
2 tablespoons low-fat mayonnaise
1/4 teaspoon dried dillweed

1. Combine brussels sprouts, seasonings, and water in a saucepan. Cover; cook to desired tenderness.
2. Remove sprouts with a slotted spoon. Stir low-cal mayonnaise and dillweed into the cooking water. Mix well with a fork or wire whisk until mixture blends and no lumps remain.
3. Cook and stir, uncovered, until liquid evaporates to a thick sauce. Pour sauce over hot brussels sprouts. Serves 3.

Serving size:	4 ounces
Exchanges:	1 vegetable
	1/2 fat
Calories:	70

CREAMY BRUSSELS SPROUTS

1 1/2 pounds brussels sprouts, washed and trimmed
2 tablespoons butter or margarine
1/4 cup lemon juice
1 cup sour cream
1/4 cup minced fresh parsley
1/2 teaspoon salt
Freshly ground black pepper
Sliced pimento-stuffed olives

1. Cut an "X" in the stem end of each sprout. Soak sprouts in cold, salted water for 10 minutes.
2. Meanwhile, melt butter in a large skillet over medium heat. Drain the sprouts; add them to the skillet. Cover and steam about 10 minutes, stirring occasionally.
3. Add the lemon juice and steam another 2 minutes; add sour cream, parsley, salt, and pepper. Heat uncovered until tender. Serve garnished with olive slices. Serves 6.

Serving size:	1/2 cup
Exchanges:	1 1/2 vegetable
	2 fat
Calories:	128

TASTY TRIMMINGS

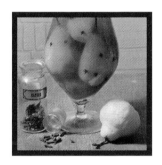

"Everything was good to eat and in

its Christmas dress."

Charles Dickens

RED TOMATO MARMALADE

2 lemons
8 ripe tomatoes, skinned and quartered
2¹/₂ cups sugar

1. Peel and juice two lemons. Cut the peel into thin shreds. Combine tomatoes, lemon peel, and lemon juice in a large saucepan. Boil uncovered for about 30 minutes. Stir in sugar and boil another 25 to 30 minutes, uncovered, until mixture begins to look like marmalade. Shake the pot several times while cooking.

2. Pour into warm, sterile jars. Cover with wax and seal tightly. Store in a cool place. Serves 6 to 8.

Serving size:	¹/₄ cup
Exchanges:	1¹/₂ fruit
Calories:	90

GREEN TOMATO MARMALADE

8 green tomatoes, skinned, quartered and ground
¹/₂ cup water
Grated peel of 2 lemons
4 to 5 1-inch pieces fresh ginger
2¹/₂ cups sugar

1. Place tomatoes in a large saucepan, add a small amount of water, the lemon peel, and ginger. Boil tomatoes until soft.

2. Pour into warm, sterile jars. Cover with wax and seal tightly. Store in a cool place. Serves 6 to 8.

Serving size:	¹/₄ cup
Exchanges:	1¹/₂ fruit
Calories:	90

PEAR RELISH

16 cups firm pears, peeled and ground
4 pounds large onions, peeled and sliced
8 green bell peppers, sliced and seeded
2 red bell peppers, sliced and seeded
2 hot peppers
12 dill pickles
1 cup salt
4 cups sugar
2 tablespoons turmeric
6 tablespoons dry mustard
2 quarts dark cider vinegar

1. Grind pears, onions, bell peppers, hot peppers, and pickles together and place in a large container. Add salt; let stand 30 minutes.

2. Meanwhile, combine sugar, turmeric, and mustard with enough vinegar to make a paste. Then place paste and remaining vinegar in a large saucepan and boil.

3. Remove from heat, then drain pear mixture and add to vinegar. Let stand for 5 minutes in the hot vinegar.

4. Pour into warm, sterile jars and seal. Serves 20 to 24.

Serving size:	1 ounce
Exchanges:	¹/₂ fruit
Calories:	30

CHERRY-VANILLA JAM

2¹/₂ cups sweet cherries, pitted
¹/₂ cup water
1 teaspoon unflavored gelatin
2 teaspoons lemon juice
2 teaspoons vanilla extract
¹/₂ teaspoon liquid artificial sweetener

1. Place cherries and water in a 1-quart saucepan. Bring to a boil, lower heat. Cover pan tightly and cook cherry mixture 5 minutes. Then stir cherries, replace cover, and cook an additional 5 minutes.

2. Pour lemon juice in small bowl. Sprinkle the gelatin over the juice.

3. When cooking is completed, remove cover. Bring fruit and juice to a boil for 1 minute. Remove mixture from heat; add gelatin and vanilla. Stir mixture until gelatin is completely dissolved. Allow mixture to cool and add artificial sweetener.

4. Pour cherry jam into sterilized jars or plastic freezer containers. Leave half an inch empty at top. Refrigerate. For long-term storage, place in freezer. Makes 2 half-pint jars.

Serving size:	2 tablespoons
Exchanges:	Free
Calories:	18

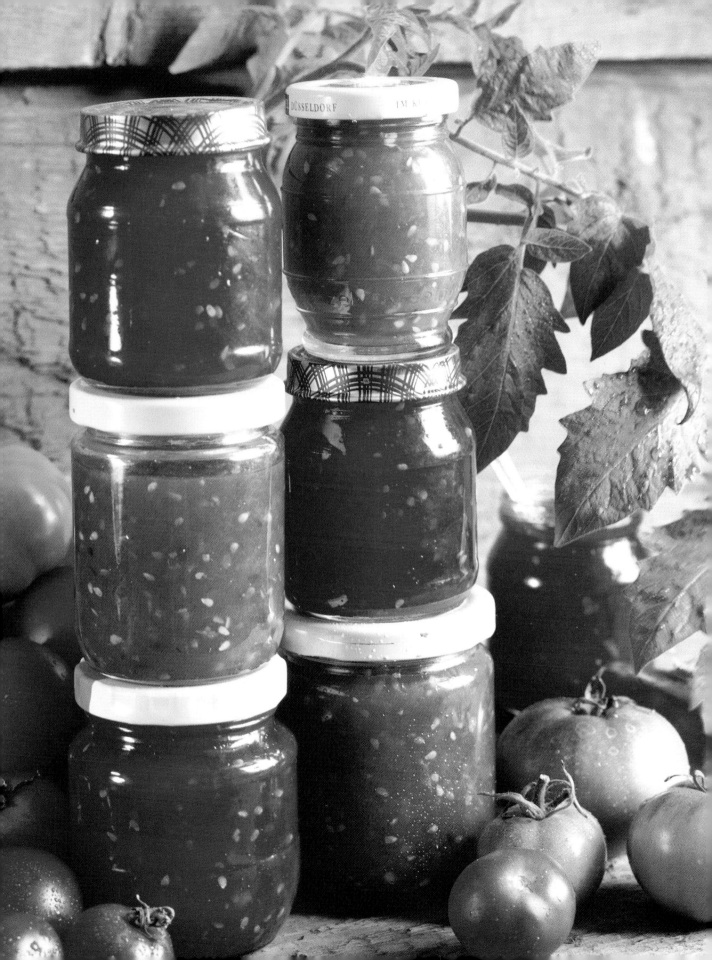

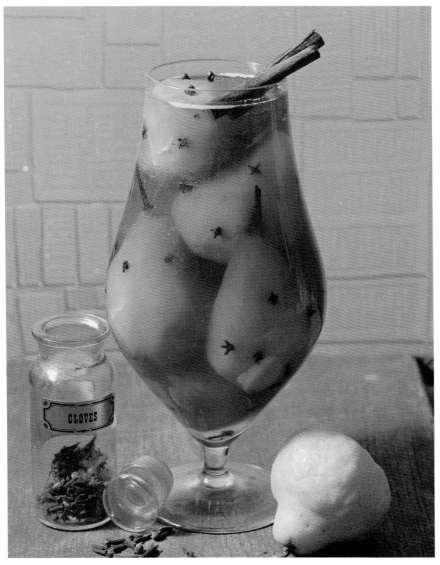

Pickled Pears

Serving size:	2¹/₂ ounces
Exchanges:	2 fruit
Calories:	120

GOOSEBERRY CONSERVE

6 cups gooseberries
1 large orange, peeled, rind grated, and
pith removed
4 cups sugar
1 cup seedless raisins

1. Clean and wash gooseberries and place in a large saucepan. Add the grated orange rind.

2. Chop orange into small pieces and add to the gooseberries. Add sugar and raisins.

3. Over low heat, stir until the sugar dissolves. Slowly bring to a boil.

4. Raise heat and cook until conserve thickens.

5. Pour into hot, sterile jars and seal. Serves 6 to 8.

Serving size:	1 ounce
Exchanges:	2 fruit
Calories:	120

PICKLED PEARS

2 cups cider vinegar
2 cups water
4 cups sugar
2 sticks cinnamon
2 1-inch pieces fresh ginger
2 to 3 tablespoons whole cloves
3 pounds pears, washed, peeled,
with stems left on

1. Put the vinegar, water, and sugar into a saucepan; add the cinnamon sticks, ginger, and 1 tablespoon of cloves. Bring slowly to a boil, and boil for 5 minutes.

2. Reduce the heat and add the pears, each stuck with 2 to 3 cloves. Poach until the pears are tender and almost transparent.

3. Pack pears into hot, sterile jars. Strain syrup and pour over pears. Seal at once. Serves 8 to 10.

DOROTHY'S SPICED CRANBERRIES

2 cups sugar
¹/₂ cup red wine vinegar
1 3-inch stick of cinnamon
³/₄ teaspoon whole cloves
4 cups fresh or frozen cranberries

1. Combine sugar, vinegar, cinnamon stick, and cloves in a large

saucepan. Bring to a boil. Add berries and cook slowly without stirring until all skins pop open.

2. Pour into warm sterile jars and seal. Serves 6 to 8.

Serving size:	1 ounces
Exchanges:	1 fruit
Calories:	60

NOTE: Chill before serving. At serving time, spoon these delicious cranberries into a serving dish.

FRENCH DRESSING

1 teaspoon Dijon mustard
2 tablespoons white wine vinegar
Salt and freshly ground black pepper
4 tablespoons olive oil

1. Mix the mustard and vinegar with salt and pepper to taste.

2. Add good olive oil and beat with a whisk until the mixture thickens. Makes $1/2$ to $3/4$ cup.

Serving size:	1 tablespoon
Exchanges:	3 fat
Calories:	135

SONYA'S RHUBARB RELISH

4 cups fresh rhubarb or frozen,
thawed rhubarb
4 cups chopped onions
$1^{1/2}$ cups cider vinegar
$1^{1/2}$ cups brown sugar, firmly packed
2 teaspoons salt
1 teaspoon allspice
1 teaspoon ground ginger
1 teaspoon ground cloves
1 teaspoon freshly ground black pepper
$3/4$ teaspoon ground cayenne pepper

1. Combine rhubarb and onions together in the vinegar-sugar mixture for 5 minutes. Add salt and spices. Simmer for 2 hours; do not boil.

2. Pour into serving dish. Cool before serving. Makes about 9 cups.

Serving size:	$1/2$ cup
Exchanges:	$1^{1/2}$ fruit
Calories:	90

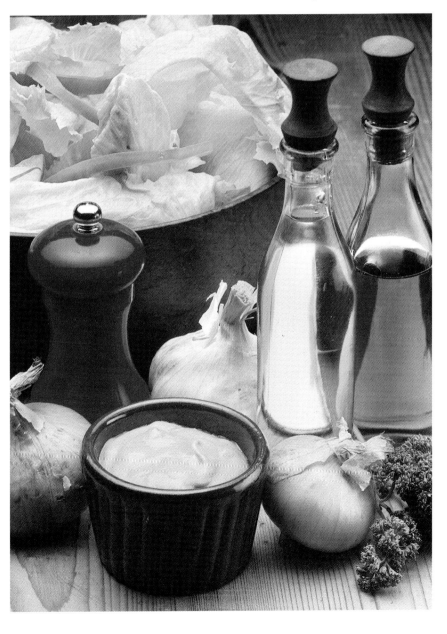

French Dressing

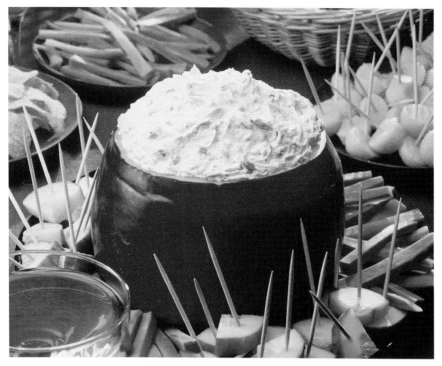

Onion Party Dip

ONION PARTY DIP

1 package French onion soup
1 cup natural yogurt
2 garlic cloves, crushed
1 tablespoon milk
Salt and freshly ground black pepper
1 teaspoon lemon juice
2 tablespoons chopped chives

1. Combine all ingredients in a bowl and stir well with a wooden spoon. Let stand for at least 3 hours before serving—this allows dip to thicken.

2. Serve in a bowl or, as in the picture, in a small scooped-out whole Edam cheese. Serves 4 to 6.

Serving size:	2 ounces
Exchanges:	Free
Calories:	20

HOLIDAY DESSERTS

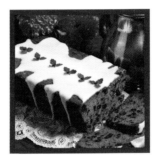

Holiday dinners would not be complete

without a sweet finale. No matter how filling

the dinner, there is always room for dessert!

CHRISTMAS TREE BREAD

FILLING
1/2 cup chopped seedless raisins
1/4 cup chopped candied cherries
1/4 cup chopped citron
1/3 cup sugar
1/3 cup boiling water
1 tablespoon lemon juice

BREAD
2 cups cake flour
2 1/2 teaspoons baking powder
1/2 teaspoon salt
3 tablespoons sugar
5 tablespoons butter or margarine
1 teaspoon lemon rind
1 large egg
1/2 cup light cream

1. Preheat oven to 400 degrees. Grease a cookie sheet.

2. Make the filling: Combine all the filling ingredients in a large saucepan. Stir over low heat until sugar has melted and mixture is well blended. Set aside to cool.

3. Make the bread: Sift the flour, baking powder, salt, and sugar together and place in a large mixing bowl. Cut in the butter and add the lemon rind. Combine the egg and cream in a small mixing bowl and beat. Stir into the flour mixture and mix to form a soft dough. Turn out onto a lightly floured board and knead for 30 seconds.

4. Divide the dough in half, and roll each half into a triangular tree-shaped piece about 1/8-inch thick. Trim off a narrow strip from the base of each triangle; cut each strip in half.

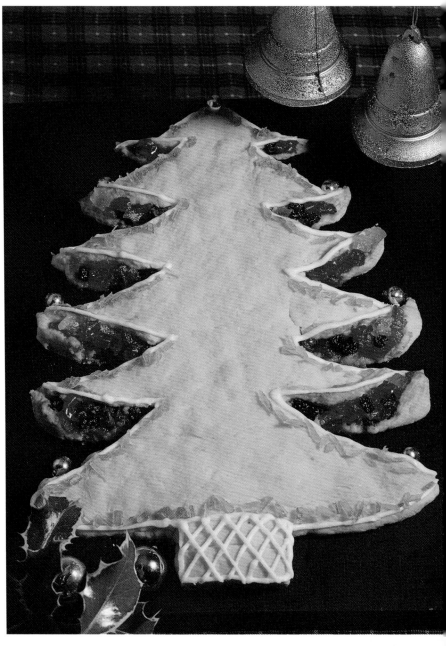

Christmas Tree B

5. Place one of the triangles on the baking sheet. Fasten two of the strips at the bottom to form the tree trunk. Spread the filling evenly over the dough, leaving a 1/4-inch edge all around. Moisten the edge, and arrange the second triangle and remaining two strips on top. Press edges firmly together.

6. Cut 4 to 5 slits on each side of the tree and twist the tips upwards to resemble branches and expose the filling. Bake for 20 minutes. Serve warm. Ice with a confectioners' sugar glaze. Serves 4 to 6.

Serving size:	2 ounces
Exchanges:	$^1/_2$ starch/bread
	2 fruit
	1 fat
Calories:	205

NEW YEAR'S PRETZELS

2 cups milk
$^1/_2$ cup butter or margarine
2 packages active dry yeast
2 teaspoons salt
$^1/_2$ cup sugar
7 to 7$^1/_2$ cups flour
2 eggs
1 cup confectioners' sugar
1 to 2 tablespoons water
1 teaspoon vanilla extract
$^1/_4$ cup chopped almonds

1. Heat milk and butter in a large saucepan until milk reaches 120 to 130 degrees. Combine yeast, salt, sugar, and 1 cup flour in a mixing bowl. Slowly beat into warm milk for 2 minutes. Add eggs and 1 cup flour. Beat for an additional 2 minutes. Stir in enough flour to form a soft dough; knead until smooth and elastic, about 6 minutes. Place dough in a greased bowl. Let rise in a warm place until doubled, about 1 hour.

2. Punch dough down and let rise again until doubled, about an hour or more.

3. Preheat oven to 375 degrees. Divide dough in half. Shape pretzel as follows: Roll dough into a rope about 30 inches long and 1$^1/_2$ inches wide. Cross the ends, leaving a large loop in the center. Flip loop back onto crossed ends to form a pretzel.

Repeat with remaining dough. Place pretzels on greased baking sheets. Let rise 15 minutes more.

4. Bake for 25 to 30 minutes, or until golden. Cool on wire racks. Mix confectioners' sugar, water, and vanilla to form a thin icing. Spread icing on pretzels and sprinkle with chopped almonds. Serves 4.

Serving size:	1$^1/_2$ ounces
Exchanges:	1 starch/bread
	1 fruit
	$^1/_2$ fat
Calories:	162

DRESDEN STOLLEN

$^1/_2$ cup raisins
$^1/_2$ cup currants
1 cup mixed candied fruit
$^1/_2$ cup candied cherries, halved
$^1/_2$ cup light rum
5 cups flour
1 package active dry yeast
$^1/_2$ teaspoon salt
1 cup sugar
1 cup milk
$^1/_2$ cup butter or margarine
2 large eggs
1 teaspoon vanilla extract
$^1/_2$ cup chopped hazelnuts (optional)
$^1/_2$ cup chopped almonds
$^1/_4$ cup butter or margarine, melted
1 cup confectioners' sugar

1. Place raisins, currants, candied fruit, and candied cherries in a large mixing bowl. Pour rum over top and let stand 1 hour. Drain fruits and reserve rum. Pat fruits dry and toss with 2 tablespoons of the flour.

2. In another large mixing bowl, combine yeast, 1 cup flour, salt, and $^3/_4$ cup sugar. Heat milk and butter in a small saucepan until milk reaches 120 to 130 degrees. Stir milk and reserved rum into flour mixture and beat for 2 minutes. Add eggs, vanilla, and an additional 1 cup flour. Beat for 2 minutes more. Add enough flour to make a soft dough.

3. Knead for 5 to 10 minutes until dough is smooth and elastic. Place dough in a lightly greased bowl. Cover and let dough rise until doubled, about 2 hours.

4. Preheat oven to 350 degrees. Punch dough down. Gently knead in candied fruits and nuts.

5. Shape the stollen: Divide dough in half. Roll one half into an 8 x 12-inch rectangle about $^1/_2$-inch thick. Brush with melted butter and sprinkle with 2 tablespoons sugar. Fold one third of the dough to the center. Repeat with other side, overlapping about 1 inch. Place on greased cookie sheet. Mold the loaf by tapering the ends to form an oval. Repeat with other half of dough. Brush top of loaves with melted butter. Let rise in warm place until doubled, about 1 hour.

6. Bake about 25 minutes until golden brown and crusty. Cool on rack. When cool, sprinkle with confectioners' sugar, or make a glaze with 2 tablespoons water and the sugar. Serves 6 to 8.

Serving size:	2 ounces
Exchanges:	1 starch/bread
	1 fruit
	1 fat
Calories:	185

GINGERBREAD CHRISTMAS COOKIES

1¼ cups sugar
⅔ cup light molasses or corn syrup
1 cup butter or margarine
⅔ cup heavy cream
1¾ tablespoons ground ginger
1 tablespoon baking soda
6 cups flour

1. Heat the sugar, molasses, and butter in a large saucepan over low heat. After butter melts, cool mixture. Stir in cream, ginger, baking soda, and flour. Let dough stand overnight.

2. Preheat oven to 400 degrees. Divide dough into thirds. Roll each piece very thin. Use a cookie cutter to cut out shapes.

3. Bake cookies on greased cookie sheets for 5 to 7 minutes. Cool on a rack. Makes 7 to 8 dozen.

Serving size:	1½ ounces
Exchanges:	2 fruit
	1 fat
Calories:	165

CHRISTMAS COOKIE VILLAGE

⅔ cup butter
1 cup sugar
¼ cup light molasses or corn syrup
⅓ cup water
½ tablespoon ground ginger
1 tablespoon ground cinnamon
½ tablespoon ground cloves
1 teaspoon powdered cardamom
½ tablespoon baking soda
3 cups flour

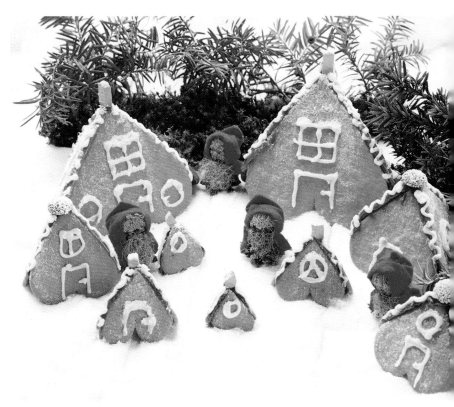

Christmas Cookie Village

1. Combine the butter, sugar, and molasses in a large mixing bowl and beat until smooth. Add the water, ginger, cinnamon, cloves, cardamom, and baking soda. Stir in enough flour to form a soft dough and fold out onto a floured bread board. Cover and let stand overnight.

2. Preheat oven to 425 degrees. Roll dough out thin. Cut out cookies with a heart-shaped cookie cutter. Bake the cookies on a greased cookie sheet in the middle of the oven for about 5 minutes. Cool them on the sheet.

3. To make the "hearts" village: Place three hearts together with their tips up to form "huts." The size of the huts can vary from tiny to extra large, depending on the size of the cutters used. Glue the sides of the hearts together by dipping the edges into sugar that has been melted in a frying pan. The sugar hardens quickly as it cools, so stick the hearts together immediately after dipping them in the sugar. The points of the hearts meet at the top of the huts. Decorate the hearts with icing, making doors and windows; use icing to hide the edges. Use colorful candy to make chimneys and other decorations. Place the huts on a bed of cotton. Sprinkle confectioners' sugar over the huts. Add Santas, greens, and other decorations.

Serving size:	1½ ounces
Exchanges:	2 fruit
	1 fat
Calories:	165

CORNFLAKE KISSES

1 egg white
1/2 cup sugar
1/4 teaspoon salt
1/2 teaspoon vanilla extract
1 cup cornflakes

1. Preheat oven to 300 degrees.
2. Beat egg white. Gradually beat in sugar, then salt and vanilla. Fold in cornflakes. Take up heaping tea-spoonfuls of mixture and push onto a well-oiled baking sheet. Bake until surface is dry (about 20 minutes). Do not brown.
3. Remove from pan with side of spatula while kisses are still warm. This freezes well. Serves 18.

Serving size:	1 kiss
Exchanges:	Free
Calories:	18

PUMPKIN BREAD

4 cups flour, unsifted
3 cups sugar
2 teaspoons baking soda
1 1/2 teaspoons salt
1 teaspoon baking powder
1 teaspoon ground cinnamon
1 teaspoon grated nutmeg
1/2 teaspoon ground cloves
1/4 teaspoon ground ginger
16-ounce can pumpkin puree or 4 cups fresh pumpkin, cooked and mashed
1 cup vegetable oil
4 large eggs
2/3 cups water

1. Preheat oven to 350 degrees.
2. Mix the dry ingredients thoroughly in a large bowl. Beat the pumpkin, oil, eggs, and water together. Stir in dry ingredients just until they are moistened. Do not over mix. Grease 2 9-inch loaf pans. Pour half of the batter into each pan.
3. Bake for 1 hour or until a toothpick inserted in the center of the loaf comes out clean. Cool on rack; remove bread from pans after 10 minutes. Serves 16.

Serving size:	1 ounce
Exchanges:	1 fruit
	1 fat
Calories:	105

Gingerbread Christmas Cookies

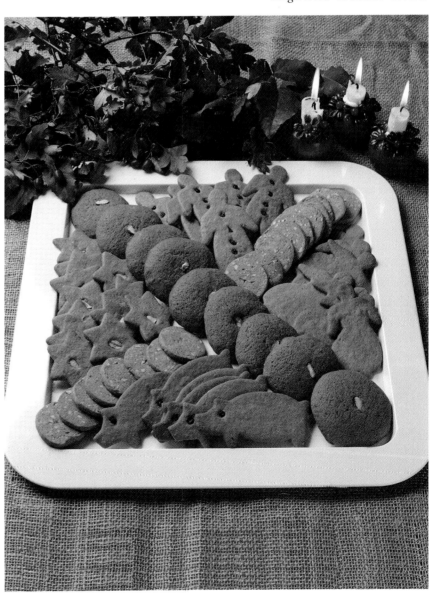

GINGERBREAD

3 cups flour
1/4 teaspoon salt
2 tablespoons ground ginger
2 teaspoons mixed pumpkin spice
2 teaspoons ground cinnamon
1/2 cup brown sugar, firmly packed
1/4 cup milk
1/2 cup light molasses
2 tablespoons dark molasses
1/2 cup butter or margarine
3 large eggs, beaten
2 teaspoons baking soda

1. Preheat oven to 375 degrees.
2. Grease sides of a 10 x 7 x 2 1/2-inch baking pan. Line with greased waxed paper.
3. In a large bowl, sift the flour, salt, and spices together. Add sugar.
4. In a small saucepan, put 3 tablespoons of milk with molasses and butter. Cook over low heat until smooth. Add the beaten eggs.
5. Stir contents of saucepan into flour mixture. Beat well.
6. Dissolve the soda in remaining milk and beat into mixture. Spread evenly into pan.
7. Bake for 50 minutes. Cool in pan; cut into squares. Serves 8.

Serving size:	1 1/2 ounces
Exchanges:	1 starch/bread
	1 fruit
Calories:	140

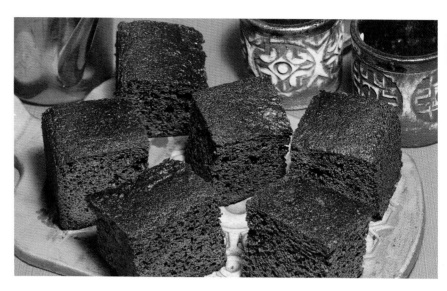

Gingerbread

DARK DATE NUT BREAD

1/2 cup boiling water
1/2 cup mixed light and dark raisins
1/2 cup chopped dates
1 1/2 tablespoons butter or margarine
3/4 teaspoon baking soda
3/4 cup plus 2 tablespoons flour, sifted
1/2 cup sugar
1/4 teaspoon salt
1 large egg
1/2 teaspoon vanilla extract
1/4 cup chopped walnuts

1. Preheat oven to 350 degrees.
2. Pour boiling water over the raisins, dates, butter, and baking soda. Let stand.
3. Mix the flour, sugar, and salt. Add fruit mixture, including water, and the remaining ingredients. Beat well. Pour batter into a greased and floured 1-pound coffee can. Bake for 60 to 70 minutes, or until done. Serves 6 to 8.

Serving size:	1 1/2 ounces
Exchanges:	1 starch/bread
	1 fruit
	1 fat
Calories:	185

MOLASSES PUMPKIN BREAD

1/3 cup butter
1 cup sugar
2 large eggs
1/2 cup light or dark molasses
1 cup canned pumpkin puree
2 cups flour
1/4 teaspoon baking powder
1 teaspoon baking soda
1/2 teaspoon pumpkin spice
1 cup coarsely chopped walnuts

1. Preheat oven to 350 degrees.
2. Cream butter in a large mixing bowl. Stir in sugar and eggs. Stir in molasses and pumpkin. Stir in the remaining ingredients and beat well. Spoon into a greased 9-inch loaf pan.

3. Bake for 1 hour or until a toothpick inserted in the center of the loaf comes out clean. Cool on a rack. Remove bread from pan after 10 minutes. Slice thinly; spread with butter or whipped cream cheese. Serves 6 to 8.

Serving size:	2 ounces
Exchanges:	2 starch/bread
	2 fat
Calories:	250

CRANBERRY-NUT BREAD

2 cups flour, sifted
1 cup sugar
1¹/2 teaspoons baking powder
¹/2 teaspoon baking soda
1 teaspoon salt
¹/4 cup butter or margarine
³/4 cup orange juice
1 tablespoon grated orange rind
1 large egg, well beaten
¹/2 cup chopped walnuts
1 or 2 cups chopped cranberries,
sprinkled with sugar

1. Preheat oven to 350 degrees.
2. Sift the flour with all the dry ingredients; cut in the shortening. Combine the orange juice and grated rind with the egg. Pour the mixture over the dry ingredients. Mix enough to dampen. Do not overmix. Fold in the chopped nuts and cranberries. Pour mixture into greased 9-inch loaf pan.
3. Bake at 350 degrees for 1 hour. Cool on rack for 5 minutes; remove from pan. Cool on rack completely. Serves 6 to 8.

Serving size:	1 ounce
Exchanges:	¹/2 starch/bread
	1 fruit
	¹/2 fat
Calories:	82

APPLE PIE

3 apples, peeled and sliced
1 bottle diet lemon soda
1 package unflavored gelatin
3 packages artificial sweetener
¹/3 cup powdered milk
Cinnamon

1. Preheat oven to 350 degrees.
2. Place apples in pie dish. Heat soda and dissolve gelatin in soda. Add 1 package sweetener. Pour over apples. Sprinkle powdered milk on top. Then sprinkle cinnamon and 2 more packages of sweetener on top. Bake for 1 hour.
3. Chill for at least 1 hour; slice and serve. Serves 6.

Serving size:	3 ounces
Exchanges:	1 fruit
Calories:	60

CUSTARD PIE

4 eggs
¹/4 teaspoon salt
¹/8 teaspoon nutmeg
1 teaspoon grated lemon peel
3 cups skim milk
32 drops liquid sugar substitute
1 teaspoon vanilla extract
1 baked 9-inch pie shell

1. Preheat oven to 450 degrees.
2. Beat eggs lightly with salt, nutmeg, and lemon peel. Stir in remaining ingredients. Set pie plate with baked shell on cookie sheet; place on rack in oven. Strain custard mixture into prepared shell.
3. Bake for 10 minutes; reduce heat to 300 degrees. Bake 45 minutes longer, or until center is almost set, but still soft. Do not overbake. Cool pie on wire rack. Cut into 8 wedges.

Serving size:	5 ounces
Exchanges:	1 medium-fat meat
	1 fruit
	1 fat
Calories:	180

PINEAPPLE CHEESE PIE

1 pound cottage cheese
1 cup pineapple pieces in juice
1 envelope gelatin
1 egg
5 packs artificial sweetener
1 teaspoon vanilla extract
1 teaspoon lemon juice
Cinnamon

1. Preheat oven to 350 degrees.
2. Put cheese and other ingredients into blender; blend until smooth. Pour into 9-inch pie plate. Sprinkle top of pie with cinnamon. Bake for 30 minutes. Cool and refrigerate. Serves 8.

Serving size:	4 ounces
Exchanges:	1 lean meat
	1 vegetable
Calories:	80

WALNUT CHEESECAKE

1/2 cup walnuts
1 cup blue cheese
3/4 cup butter
*1/2 to 2/3 cup firm whipped or solid
cream cheese*
2/3 cup half and half cream
Green and purple grapes
Chives for garnish

1. Remove several of the more decorative walnuts for the garnish. Finely chop or grind the rest of the walnuts. Add them to the blue cheese and 7 tablespoons of the butter. Make into a soft mixture.

2. Warm the cream cheese and the cream and mix in the rest of the butter. Remove from the heat as soon as the cheese has melted. Place cut greased baking paper on the bottom of small springform pan. Spread half of the cheese mixture, about 1/2 inch thick, into the pan. Cover with the soft blue-cheese mixture. Cover this with the rest of the cream cheese mixture. Even the top with a small, warmed spatula. Decorate with the reserved walnuts. Refrigerate for at least 24 hours.

3. Remove the edge and bottom of the pan when the cake is cold. Take the cake out of the refrigerator and serve it at room temperature. Garnish with grapes. Make division lines on the cake with chives.

NOTE: This cake tastes best when it is two days old and not served too cold. Serves 8.

Serving size:	1 slice
Exchanges:	2 medium-fat meat
	1/2 fruit
	8 fat
Calories:	540

SPICE MERINGUES

1 egg white
Pinch of salt
1/2 teaspoon ground cinnamon
Pinch of ground cloves
1/4 cup sugar
1/4 cup finely chopped nuts
*1/2 cup natural (unsweetened) wheat
and barley "nut" cereal*

1. Preheat oven to 300 degrees.

2. Beat egg white with salt until it forms soft peaks. Mix the cinnamon, cloves, and sugar together. Gradually beat into egg white until very stiff. Fold in nuts and cereal. Drop by teaspoonfuls onto cookie tins lined with aluminum foil. Bake 1 to 1 1/4 hours. Then turn off oven and allow the meringues to cool slowly.

3. When cool, peel off foil. Store in tightly covered container to protect from dampness. Serves 30.

Serving size:	2 meringues
Exchanges:	Free
Calories:	20

Walnut Cheesecake

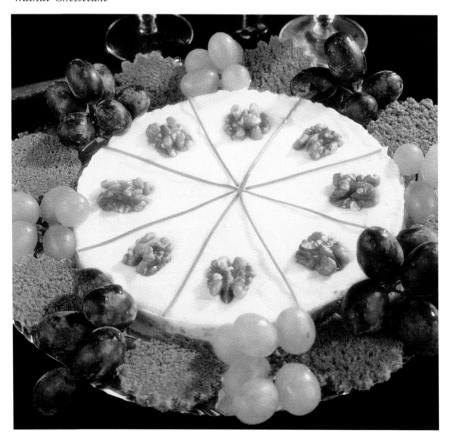

CHOCOLATE MERINGUE SQUARES

CHOCOLATE BATTER
*8 tablespoons butter or margarine,
softened*
1/3 cup sugar
3 egg yolks
2/3 cup flour
*3 tablespoons cocoa, unsweetened
powdered*
2 teaspoons baking powder
1/4 cup milk

MERINGUE BATTER
3 egg whites
3/4 cup sugar
1/2 cup chopped hazelnuts

1. Preheat oven to 350 degrees.
2. Cover a baking sheet with baking parchment paper or wax paper. Grease paper with 1 tablespoon butter.
3. Make chocolate batter. Combine remaining butter and sugar and beat until airy. Add the egg yolks, one at a time. Combine flour, cocoa, and baking powder in small mixing bowl. Alternate adding this mixture and the milk to the egg yolk mixture. Spread the batter onto the baking sheet with rubber spatula.
4. Make meringue batter: Place egg whites in mixing bowl and whip into dry peaks. Gradually beat in the sugar until soft peaks form. Spread the meringue batter over the chocolate batter. Sprinkle with the nuts.
5. Bake for 20 to 25 minutes. Cool cake on rack. Cut into squares with a sharp knife. Make: 20 to 25 squares.

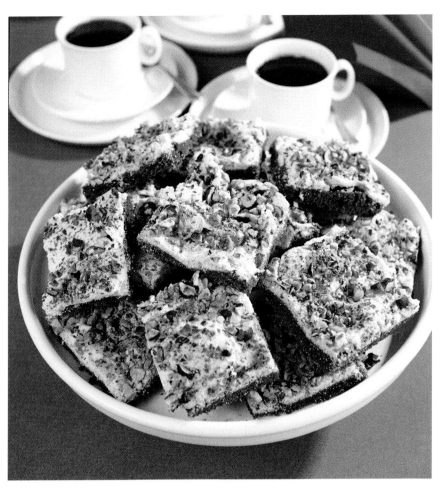

Chocolate Meringue Squares

Serving size:	1 ounce
Exchanges:	1 starch/bread
	1 fat
Calories:	125

PECAN PIE

5 large eggs
3/4 cup sugar
1 1/2 cups dark corn syrup
1 1/2 cups pecans, halved
3/4 teaspoon salt
2 teaspoons vanilla extract
Unbaked 9-inch pastry shell
Whipped cream for garnish

1. Preheat oven to 325 degrees.
2. Place eggs in a large mixing bowl and beat slightly. Add sugar, syrup, nuts, salt, and vanilla. Mix until blended.
3. Pour into pie shell. Bake for 50 minutes. Remove from oven and cool. Serve with whipped cream. Serves 6.

Serving size:	2 ounce slice
Exchanges:	1 starch/bread
	1 fruit
	1 fat
Calories:	185

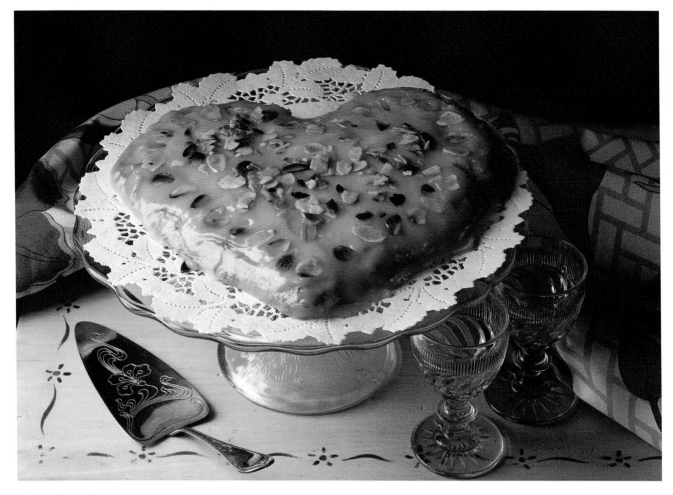

Alexander Cake

ALEXANDER CAKE

CAKE
1/4 cup whole almonds
5 egg whites
3/4 cup sugar

CUSTARD CREAM
5 egg yolks
1 1/4 cups heavy cream
3/4 cup sugar
1 teaspoon cornstarch
2 teaspoons rum
1 cup toasted sliced almonds
for garnish

1. Preheat oven to 350 degrees.
2. Grind the almonds. Whip the egg whites in a large mixing bowl until stiff. Fold in the almonds and sugar. Spread the batter into 2 equal-sized heart-shaped layers on greased cookie sheet. Bake for 15 minutes.

3. Make the custard cream: Combine the egg yolks, cream, sugar, and cornstarch in the top of a double boiler. Let the custard cream cook slowly over boiling water for 10 to 15 minutes or until it thickens. Stir constantly. Stir in the rum, then cool.

4. Frost top of one layer with half the custard cream. Place the second layer on top and spread with remaining cream. Garnish with almonds. Serves 8 to 10.

Serving size:	3 ounce slice
Exchanges:	3 starch/bread
	3 fat
Calories:	375

SUGAR CAKE

1 1/4 cups flour
3/4 cup sugar
1/2 teaspoon vanilla extract extract
1 teaspoon baking powder
2 eggs
1/4 cup water
2/3 cup margarine or butter

1. Preheat oven to 350 degrees. Grease a 1 1/2-quart round cake pan

and dust with bread crumbs or flour.

2. Measure all cake ingredients into food processor, heavy duty blender or electric mixer bowl.

3. Divide the margarine into 6 to 8 pieces before adding. Mix for 20 to 30 seconds.

4. Pour the batter into a 1$\frac{1}{2}$-quart prepared pan. Bake in the lower half of the oven for about 40 minutes. Let cake cool before removing from pan. Serves 8.

Serving size:	3 ounce slice
Exchanges:	1 starch/bread
	2 fruit
	3 fat
Calories:	335

HONEY ORANGE HIGH-FIBER BREAD PUDDING

4 slices high-fiber bread, diced (can be slightly stale)

6 tablespoons raisins
$\frac{1}{2}$ teaspoon cinnamon or pumpkin pie spice
3 eggs
$\frac{1}{4}$ cup honey
1$\frac{1}{2}$ cups orange juice
1 teaspoon vanilla extract
$\frac{1}{4}$ teaspoon salt

1. Preheat oven to 350 degrees.

2. Spray a small nonstick loaf pan with cooking spray. Combine bread with raisins in loaf pan. Sprinkle with cinnamon or pumpkin pie spice and mix well.

3. Combine remaining ingredients in blender, processor or electric mixer bowl and beat until blended. Pour over bread.

4. Set the loaf pan in a larger pan; add boiling water to the larger pan. Slide the pan into the oven. Bake 35 to 45 minutes, until a knife inserted in the center comes out clean. Serves 6.

Serving size:	4 ounces
Exchanges:	1$\frac{1}{2}$ starch/bread
	1 fat
Calories:	165

APPLE CRUMBLE

2 pounds firm cooking apples, peeled, cored and sliced
2 teaspoons lemon juice
$\frac{1}{4}$ teaspoon grated nutmeg
$\frac{1}{2}$ teaspoon ground cinnamon
1 cup sugar
2 tablespoons water
$\frac{3}{4}$ cup flour
$\frac{1}{8}$ teaspoon salt
$\frac{1}{4}$ cup butter or margarine
$\frac{1}{4}$ cup chopped nuts

1. Preheat oven to 350 degrees.

2. Combine the apples, lemon juice, spices, and half of the sugar. Toss together, and place in greased 2-quart baking dish. Add 2 tablespoons of water.

3. Sift the flour with salt, cut in the butter, and add the remaining sugar and the nuts. Sprinkle over top of the apples.

4. Bake for about 45 minutes. Serves 4 to 6.

Serving size:	3 ounces
Exchanges:	2 fruit
	1 fat
Calories:	165

Sugar Cake

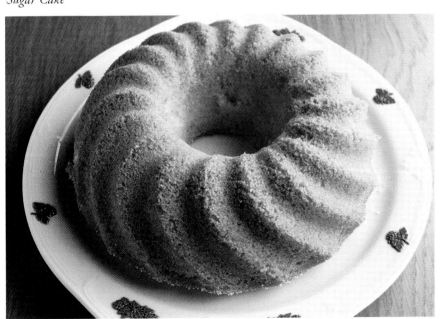

CINNAMON CAKE

CAKE
7 tablespoons butter
3/4 cup sugar
3 large eggs
1 2/3 cups flour
2 teaspoons baking powder
1/2 teaspoon vanilla extract
3/4 cup sour cream

FILLING
About 1/4 cup sugar
1 teaspoon cinnamon

1. Preheat oven to 350 degrees.
2. Grease 1 1/2-quart baking dish and dust with flour.
3. Combine butter and sugar in a large mixing bowl. Beat until light and fluffy. Add the eggs, one at a time, beating constantly.
4. Blend the flour and baking powder. Stir the vanilla into the sour cream. Combine sugar and cinnamon. Alternate adding the flour mixture and the sour cream to the butter mixture.
5. Pour half of the batter into a baking dish. Sprinkle half of the sugar and cinnamon mixture on top. Cover with rest of the batter. Top with remaining sugar and cinnamon.
6. Bake for about 1 hour; cover cake with aluminum foil if it browns too much. Serves 6 to 8.

Serving size:	2 ounce slice
Exchanges:	1 starch/bread
	1 fruit
	2 fat
Calories:	230

OLD-FASHIONED GINGERBREAD CAKE

About 2 cups flour
1 teaspoon baking soda
3 large eggs
1 1/4 cups sugar
2/3 cup butter, melted
1 tablespoon ground ginger
1 tablespoon ground cinnamon
1 tablespoon ground cloves
2/3 cup lingonberry or cranberry jam
2/3 cup sour cream

1. Preheat oven to 350 degrees.
2. Grease 2-quart oblong baking dish and dust with bread crumbs or flour.
3. Blend the flour and baking soda and set aside.
4. Combine eggs and sugar in a large mixing bowl and beat until light and airy. Stir in the butter, spices, jam, sour cream, and the flour/baking soda mixture. Pour the batter into baking dish.
5. Bake about 1 hour or until toothpick inserted in center of cake comes out clean. Serves 12 to 14.

Serving size:	2 ounce slice
Exchanges:	1 starch/bread
	1 fruit
	2 fat
Calories:	230

SAND CAKE

3/4 to 1 cup butter or margarine
1 2/3 cups potato flour, or 3 1/3 cups regular flour
1 teaspoon baking powder
3 large eggs
3/4 cup sugar
2 tablespoons brandy

1. Preheat oven to 350 degrees.
2. Grease a 1 1/2 quart baking dish and dust with bread crumbs or flour.
3. Combine butter, flour, and baking powder in a large mixing bowl. Beat until very light and fluffy.
4. Mix eggs and sugar in another bowl. Beat until light and airy. Add to butter mixture. Spoon in brandy. Pour the batter into baking dish.
5. Bake for about 40 minutes. Serves 8.

Serving size:	2 ounce slice
Exchanges:	1 starch/bread
	1 1/2 fruit
	2 fat
Calories:	260

*Cinnamon Cake, Sand Cake, and
Old-fashioned Gingerbread Cake*

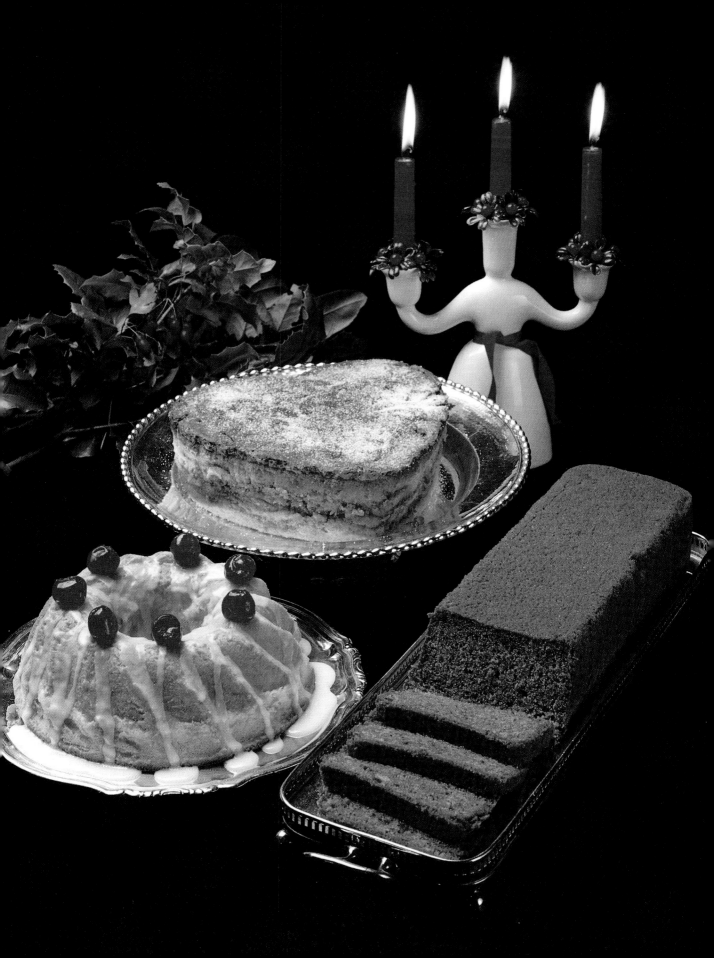

FORGOTTEN MERINGUE CAKE

CAKE
5 egg whites
1 1/4 cups sugar
1/2 teaspoon baking powder

FILLING
Ice cream
Strawberries

1. Preheat oven to 450 degrees.
2. Beat egg whites until stiff. Add sugar and baking powder, beating continuously. Pour batter into a greased ring pan. Smooth top slightly. When oven has reached 450 degrees, turn it off. Then place meringue in oven. Leave for about 9 hours or overnight.
3. Put on serving dishes with strawberries and ice cream. Serves 8 to 10.

Serving size:	1 serving
Exchanges:	1 starch/bread
	2 fruit
	1 fat
Calories:	245

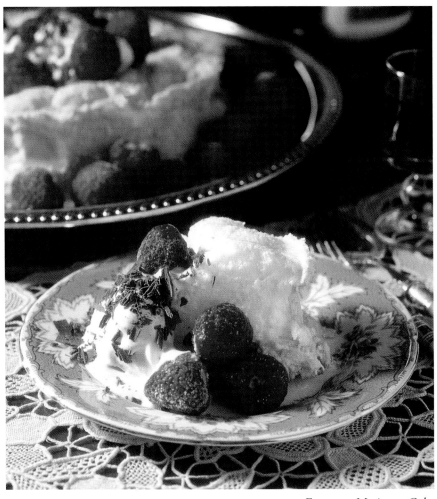

Forgotten Meringue Cake

YULE LOG

CAKE
3 large eggs
1/2 cup sugar
1/2 cup plus 1 tablespoon flour
1 tablespoon unsweetened cocoa

FILLING
3/4 cup butter, softened
1 1/2 cups confectioners' sugar
1/2 teaspoon vanilla extract extract
1 tablespoon unsweetened cocoa

1. Preheat oven to 425 degrees. Grease and line with wax paper a shallow 9 x 12-inch jelly roll or baking pan.
2. Combine eggs and sugar in a large mixing bowl. Whisk until thick and pale. Sift the flour and cocoa together three times, and fold gently into the egg mixture. Pour batter into the pan and bake for 7 to 10 minutes.
3. Meanwhile, lay a sheet of waxed paper on a flat surface and sprinkle with confectioners' sugar. When the center of the cake feels firm, turn out onto the paper, trim edges, lay a second sheet of paper on top, and roll up firmly. Chill in refrigerator.
4. To make the filling: Combine butter, sugar, and vanilla in a mixing bowl and cream. When the cake is cold, unroll gently and spread half the filling on the inside; roll up again.
5. Add cocoa to remaining filling and frost the cake. Take a fork to mark "bark" in frosting by running the tines down the log. Decorate as desired and chill until serving. Serves 8.

NOTE: Make this Yule Log no earlier than the day before serving. Decorate log with green and red frosting.

Serving size:	2 ounce slice
Exchanges:	1 starch/bread
	1½ fruit
	2 fat
Calories:	260

APPLE RICE

½ cup round-grained rice
1 cup water
½ teaspoon salt
3 sour apples
2 tablespoons sugar
½ cup heavy cream, whipped (can be omitted if the rice is to be eaten warm)
1 ounce roasted sliced almonds
Cinnamon

1. Boil the rice in the water for about 10 minutes.
2. Peel the apples, if you wish. Carefully remove all of the core. Cut the apples into small cubes. Stir the fruit and sugar into the rice. Boil for 5 minutes, then let stand for 5 minutes. Let the rice cool.
3. Whip the cream and stir it into the apple rice. Sprinkle roasted almonds on top of the rice. Spice with cinnamon. Add milk if the rice is warm. Serves 4.

Serving size:	4 ounces
Exchanges:	1 starch/bread
	½ fruit
	2 fat
Calories:	200

CHOCOLATE MOUSSE

2 envelopes unflavored gelatin
1½ cups skim milk, divided
1 cup low-fat cottage cheese
3 envelopes light cocoa mix
2 eggs, separated
¼ cup sugar

1. Soften gelatin in ½ cup milk. Heat and stir until gelatin is completely dissolved. Pour into blender container with remaining milk, cheese, cocoa mix, and egg yolks. Blend until smooth. Chill until thick.
2. Beat egg whites until stiff. Gradually beat in sugar. Fold in cocoa mixture. Chill until firm in a serving bowl, or in 6 individual dessert cups. Serves 6.

Serving size:	4 ounces
Exchanges:	1 starch/bread
	1 lean meat
	½ fruit
Calories:	165

Apple Rice

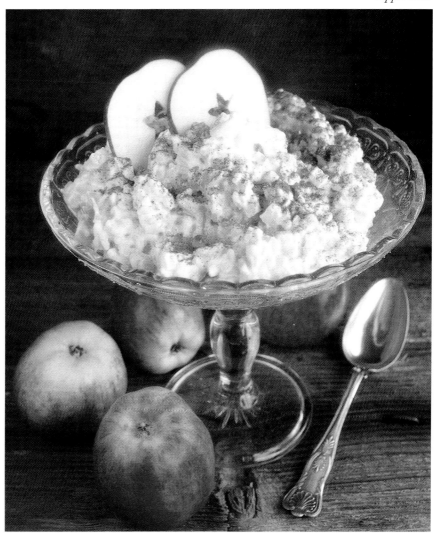

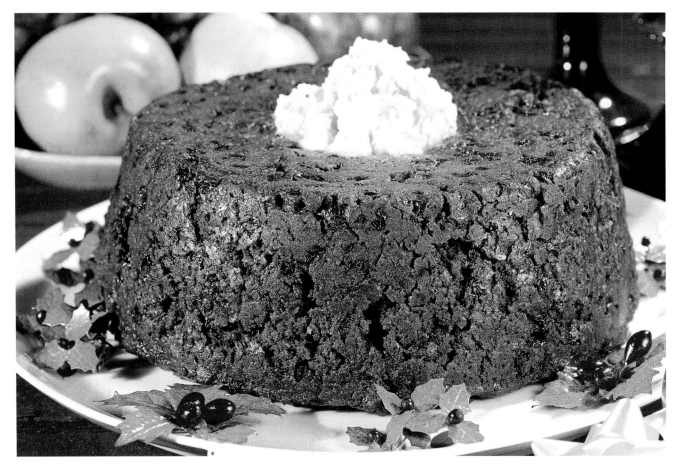

Special Christmas Pudding

SPECIAL CHRISTMAS PUDDING

1 cup flour
1 teaspoon baking powder
1 teaspoon pumpkin pie spice mixture
1/8 teaspoon salt
3/4 cup soft bread crumbs
3/4 cup chopped suet
1/2 cup brown sugar, firmly packed
5 tablespoons raisins
5 tablespoons currants
2 large cooking apples, peeled, cored, and finely chopped
5 tablespoons chopped citron
1/4 cup molasses
1/2 cup milk
2 tablespoons brandy or rum

1. Grease a 2-quart ring mold and sprinkle with brown sugar.

2. Sift the flour, baking powder, spice, and salt together and place in a large mixing bowl. Stir in bread crumbs, suet, sugar, and fruits.

3. Combine the molasses with the milk and brandy. Stir into pudding and mix well.

4. Turn into mold. Cover with greased wax paper and then with foil. Place mold on a trivet in a heavy pan over 1 inch of water. Cover and steam for 4 hours, adding water as needed.

5. Remove the paper, re-cover, and store in a dry place. Before serving, steam another 1 1/2 hours. Serves 5 to 6.

Serving size:	2 ounces
Exchanges:	2 fruit
	2 fat
Calories:	210

BAKED PEARS

6 medium Bartlett pears
6 whole cloves
1 1/2 cups wine
3/4 cup sugar
3/4 cup water

1. Preheat oven to 400 degrees.

2. Pierce bottom of pear with a clove. Place unpeeled pears into a 2-quart baking dish. Combine the remaining ingredients and pour over

the pears. Cover with foil and bake for about 30 minutes or until done. Baste occasionally. Serves 6.

Serving size:	¹/2 pear
Exchanges:	1 fruit
Calories:	60

SAFFRON ADVENT CAKE

2 cups flour
3 teaspoons baking powder
³/4 cup sugar
7 tablespoons butter
²/3 cup milk
1 large egg
¹/4 teaspoon saffron, crumbled
3 or 4 large apples, thinly sliced
Several pinches of sugar and dabs of butter

1. Preheat oven to 425 degrees.
2. Grease springform baking pan, and dust with bread crumbs or flour.
3. Combine the flour, baking powder, and sugar in a large mixing bowl. Crumble the butter into mixture until it is grainy.
4. Beat together milk, egg and saffron in large mixing bowl. Pour into the flour mixture. Stir quickly into a dough and place in pan. Stick apple slices into the surface of the dough. Sprinkle the whole surface with sugar and dot with butter.
5. Bake for 25 to 30 minutes. Serves 10.

Serving size:	2 ounce slice
Exchanges:	1 starch/bread
	1 fruit
	2 fat
Calories:	230

ORANGE-NUT RING

³/4 cup butter, softened
3 large eggs
1 cup sugar
Rind of 1 large or 2 small oranges, grated
¹/4 to ¹/3 cup pecans, chopped
1 cup flour

1. Preheat oven to 350 degrees.
2. Grease a 9-inch ring cake pan and sprinkle with bread crumbs.
3. Place butter in large mixing bowl and beat until light. Combine the eggs and sugar in a large mixing bowl. Beat until light and airy. Stir the mixture into butter then carefully stir in orange rind, pecans, and flour. Pour into prepared pan.
4. Bake for 30 to 40 minutes, or until the cake feels dry. Enhance the flavor of this cake by moistening with a sugar syrup of confectioners' sugar flavored with squeezed orange juice or orange liqueur.
5. Make the sugar syrup: Boil ¹/2 cup sugar in 2 cups water until syrupy. Prick the cake and spoon the liquid over the cake. Serves 6 to 8.

Serving size:	2 ounce slice
Exchanges:	1 starch/bread
	1 fruit
	2 fat
Calories:	230

Saffron Advent Cake and Orange-Nut Ring

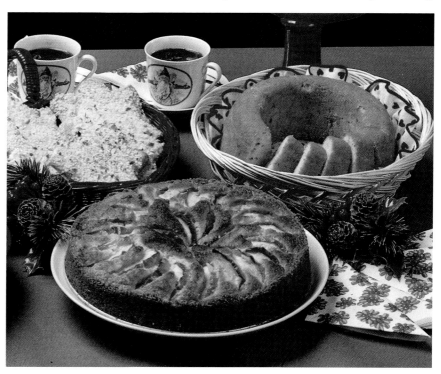

FRUIT SAVARIN

CAKE
5 tablespoons almonds, slivered
1 cup milk
3 cakes compressed yeast
4 cups flour
1 cup butter or margarine, softened
3/4 cup sugar
5 large eggs
1 teaspoon salt

FILLING
1 cup peach slices
1 cup apricot halves
1 cup pineapple rings
1 cup pitted cherries
Juice of half a lemon
1/4 cup honey
2 to 3 tablespoons light rum

1. Preheat the oven to 400 degrees.
2. Grease a 9-inch fluted tube pan and sprinkle with almonds.
3. Scald milk; cool slightly till lukewarm. Pour over the yeast in a large mixing bowl. Stir until dissolved. Sift in 1 cup of the flour, beat well. Leave in a warm place until doubled.
4. Meanwhile, place butter in a large mixing bowl and beat with sugar until fluffy. Beat in eggs, 1 at a time. Add the remaining flour and salt.
5. Combine the two mixtures. Beat together and pour into pan. Leave in a warm place until almost doubled.
6. Bake for 50 to 60 minutes.
7. Make the syrup: Drain the fruits, and put 1 1/2 cups of the syrup into a large saucepan with lemon juice and honey. Boil for 5 minutes; add rum to taste.
8. When the savarin is done, turn out onto a rack. Prick all over with a fine skewer. Pour all but 1/4 cup hot syrup over top. Fill the center with the fruit. Boil the remaining syrup until reduced and thick. Pour over the fruit. Serves 6 to 8.

Serving size:	2 ounce slice
Exchanges:	2 fruit
	1 fat
Calories:	165

CHRISTMAS RING

CAKE
1/2 cup cake flour, minus 2 teaspoons
2 teaspoons cornstarch
2 tablespoons sugar
5 egg whites
3 tablespoons clear honey
1/8 teaspoon salt
1 teaspoon cream of tartar
1 teaspoon vanilla extract extract

FROSTING
1 pound sugar cubes
1/2 cup water
2 egg whites

1. Preheat oven to 250 degrees.
2. Make the cake: Sift the flour and cornstarch together at least 4 times. Add the sugar and sift again. Place in a large mixing bowl.
3. Place the egg whites in a large mixing bowl. Beat the egg whites until stiff. Add honey, salt, and cream of tartar. Whisk again until stiff but not dry.
4. Add vanilla. Fold in flour very carefully, a spoonful at a time. Carefully scoop batter into an ungreased 9-inch angel cake tube pan

Fruit Savarin

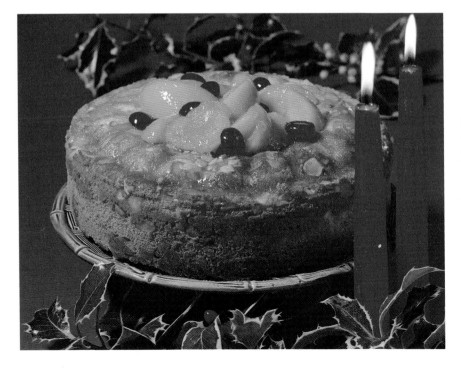

with removable sides.

5. Bake at 250 degrees for 35 minutes; raise temperature to 325 degrees and bake 10 minutes longer. To test for doneness, press lightly on top to check if firm. Remove from oven, invert pan. Allow to cool before removing from pan.

6. Make the frosting: Place sugar and water in a small saucepan and cook over low heat until sugar has melted. Then bring to boil at 238 degrees, or until the "soft ball" stage.

7. Remove at once from heat, cool slightly. Then pour very slowly and steadily into the egg whites, stirring gently to incorporate. Drizzle over the cake and carefully form peaks with a broad spatula. Set aside to cool completely. Serves 8 to 9.

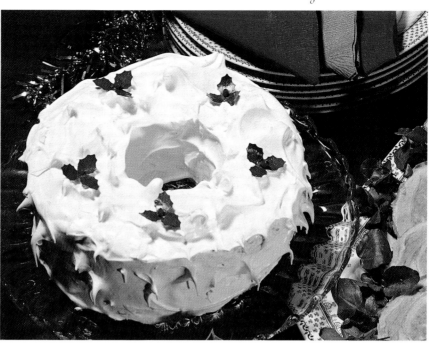

Christmas Ring

CHRISTMAS RING

Serving size:	2 ounce slice
Exchanges:	1 starch/bread
	1 fruit
Calories:	140

FROSTING

Serving size:	2 ounce slice
Exchanges:	1 fruit
Calories:	60

LIME DESSERT FLUFF

¹/₂ teaspoon unflavored gelatin
1 teaspoon sugar
¹/₂ cup evaporated low-fat milk
4 to 5 drops green food color
1 teaspoon bottled sweetened lime juice
1 teaspoon grated lime peel

1. In saucepan combine gelatin and sugar. Stir in evaporated milk. Stir over low heat until gelatin dissolves. Tint to desired color with food color. Freeze until icy cold.

2. Whip to stiff peaks. Beat in lime juice. Use as topping over dessert and sprinkle with grated lime peel. Makes about 2 cups.

Serving size:	4 tablespoons
Exchanges:	Free
Calories:	16

RASPBERRY PARFAIT

1 tablespoon instant tapioca
1 cup milk
1 egg, separated
¹/₄ teaspoon vanilla extract
¹/₈ teaspoon salt
1 cup raspberries, unsweetened, canned or frozen

1. Cook the tapioca and milk in a double boiler until the tapioca becomes transparent.

2. Beat the egg yolk, add the milk and tapioca mixture to it, and return to double boiler. Cook until the mixture thickens. This requires frequent stirring. Cool slightly; add vanilla, salt, and raspberries.

3. Beat the egg white until it becomes very stiff and fold into tapioca mixture. Chill and divide into two equal portions, piling each into a parfait glass.

Serving size:	5 ounces
Exchanges:	1 starch/bread
	1 fruit
	1 fat
Calories:	185

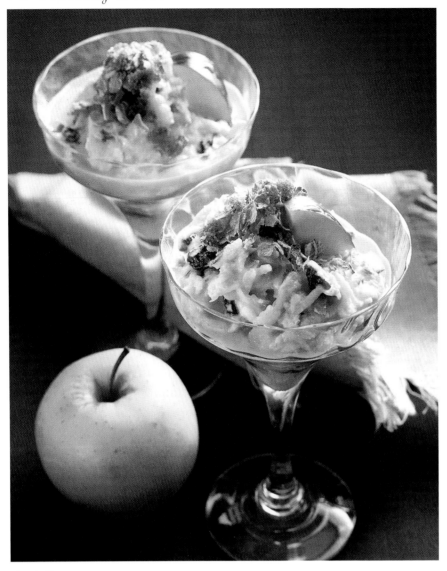

Apple Yummy

BAKED APPLES WITH NUTMEG SAUCE

4 apples, washed and cored
1/8 teaspoon liquid sweetener, more if desired
1/2 teaspoon cinnamon
1 cup water

NUTMEG SAUCE
1 1/2 tablespoons cornstarch
1/2 teaspoon nutmeg
Dash of salt
3 tablespoons artificial sweetener
1 1/2 cups water
1 tablespoon butter
1 teaspoon vanilla extract

1. Preheat oven to 350 degrees.
2. Pare and core apples, standing them in a shallow baking pan. Mix sweetener, cinnamon and water. Pour over the apples.
3. Bake at 350 degrees for about 1 hour. If desired, apples can be frozen after baking for future use.
4. Combine the cornstarch, nutmeg, and salt. Add sweetener and a small amount of water to make a smooth paste. Add the remaining water. Cook over low heat stirring constantly until mixture is thickened. Remove from heat. Add the butter and vanilla.
5. Serve warm or cool over the baked apple using 1/4 cup per apple. Serves 4.

APPLE	
Serving size:	1 apple
Exchanges:	1 fruit
Calories:	60

NUTMEG SAUCE	
Serving size:	1 1/2 tablespoons
Exchanges:	Free
Calories:	4

APPLE YUMMY

3 bitter apples
1/3 cup raisins
1 1/4 cups sour cream or yogurt, cold
3 tablespoons frozen orange juice, partially thawed
2 tablespoons granola

1. Peel and grate the apples. Mix the grated apples and the raisins with the cold sour cream. Quickly fold in the partially thawed orange juice (it should still be slightly icy) with the sour cream mixture. Spoon into tall glasses.
2. Sprinkle with granola. Serve immediately. Serves 2 to 3.

Serving size:	3 ounces
Exchanges:	1 starch/bread
Calories:	80

SILVER APPLES

4 ripe tart cooking apples, peeled
1 lemon, halved
²/3 cup apricot jam
¹/4 cup water
2 tablespoons sugar
¹/2 teaspoon vanilla extract
2 tablespoons almond extract

1. Preheat oven to 425 degrees.

2. Rub surfaces of apples with lemon to prevent discoloring.

3. Place the apricot jam into a medium saucepan. Add water and sugar. Boil until mixture thickens. Add the vanilla and almond extract.

4. Tear off 4 sheets of aluminum foil. Shape a strip of foil into 4 deep bowls. Place one apple in each, and divide the sauce equally over the apples. Seal the aluminum closed tightly.

5. Bake for about 25 minutes. Serves 4.

NOTE: For a variation of this glamorous dessert, prepare and serve pears in the same way as the apples. Serve with vanilla or other flavor ice cream.

Serving size:	1 apple
Exchanges:	4 fruit
Calories:	240

COFFEE CONFECTION

1¹/2 envelopes unflavored gelatin
1¹/2 cups water
1 cup milk
³/4 cup sugar
¹/4 teaspoon salt
2 tablespoons instant coffee granules
3 large eggs, separated
1 teaspoon vanilla extract

1. Combine the gelatin, water, milk, sugar, salt, and coffee in the top of a double boiler over medium heat. Stir until the gelatin has dissolved and the mixture is almost boiling.

2. Add the egg yolks, lower the heat, and cook until the mixture is thick enough to coat the back of a spoon.

3. Remove from the heat. Add the vanilla, and chill until the mixture is syrupy. Beat the egg whites until stiff, and fold into the mixture.

4. Pour into sherbet glasses. Chill until firm and garnish with whipped cream, if desired. Serves 4.

Serving size:	2 ounces
Exchanges:	1 starch/bread
Calories:	80

Silver Apples

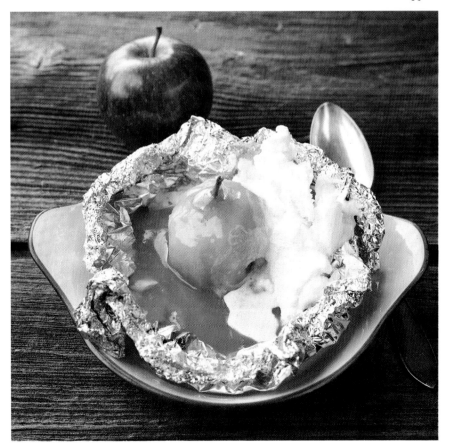

CHRISTMAS FRUIT LOAF

4 cups cake flour
1 teaspoon baking powder
1/2 teaspoon ground cloves
1/2 teaspoon ground cinnamon
1/4 teaspoon ground nutmeg
1/4 teaspoon ground mace
2 cups butter or margarine
2 1/4 cups brown sugar, firmly packed
10 large eggs, beaten
1 1/2 cups candied or maraschino cherries
1 1/2 cups candied pineapples
2 1/2 cups dates, chopped
2 1/2 cups seedless raisins
2 1/2 cups currants
2 cups mixed candied orange and lemon peel
1 1/4 cups walnuts, chopped
1 cup honey
1 cup light molasses
1/4 cup cider
1/4 cup brandy or rum

1. Preheat oven to 250 degrees.
2. Grease 3 loaf pans (10 x 5 x 3-inches); line with greased wax paper.
3. Sift together the flour, baking powder, and spices three times and place in large mixing bowl.
4. Cream the butter in a large mixing bowl, and gradually beat in sugar until light and fluffy. Add the eggs, fruit, candied peels, nuts, honey, molasses, cider, and brandy.
5. Add the flour and spice mixture gradually, beating after each addition. Place in the loaf pans. Bake for 3 1/2 to 4 hours. Serves 8 to 10.

NOTE: To keep extra or leftover fruit loaf, wrap tightly in aluminum foil. Then freeze or refrigerate.

Serving size:	1 ounce slice
Exchanges:	1 1/2 fruit
Calories:	90

PLUM PUDDING

1 1/2 cups currants
2 cups seedless black raisins
2 cups golden raisins
3/4 cup finely chopped candied mixed fruit peel
3/4 cup finely chopped candied cherries
1 cup almonds, blanched, slivered
1 large tart apple, peeled, quartered, cored, and coarsely chopped
1 small carrot, scraped and coarsely chopped
2 tablespoons orange rind, finely grated
2 teaspoons lemon rind, finely grated
1/2 pound beef suet, finely chopped
2 cups flour
4 cups bread crumbs, fresh
1 cup dark brown sugar, firmly packed
1 teaspoon ground allspice
1 teaspoon salt
6 large eggs
1 cup brandy
1/3 cup fresh orange juice
1/4 cup fresh lemon juice
1/2 cup brandy, for flaming (optional)

1. Combine the currants, raisins, candied fruit peel, cherries, almonds, apple, carrot, orange and lemon rind, and beef suet in a large mixing bowl. Stir them with a spoon until well mixed. Stir in the flour, bread crumbs, brown sugar, allspice, and salt.

2. In a separate bowl, beat the eggs until frothy. Stir in 1 cup brandy and the juices. Pour liquid over the fruit mixture. Stir vigorously until all ingredients are blended. Drape a dampened kitchen towel over the bowl and refrigerate for at least 12 hours.

Christmas Fruit Loaf

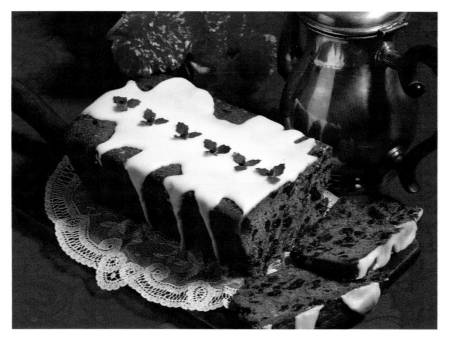

3. Spoon mixture into 4 plain molds (1 quart each), filling them to within 2 inches of their tops. Cover each mold with a strip of greased foil, turning the edges down and pressing the foil tightly around the sides to secure it. Drape a dampened kitchen towel over each mold and tie it in place around the sides. Bring 2 opposite corners of the towel up to the top and knot them in the center of the mold, then bring up the remaining 2 corners and knot them the same way.

4. Place the molds in a large stockpot and pour in enough water to reach about three-quarters of the way up their sides. Bring the water to boil; cover pot tightly. Reduce heat to lowest point; steam puddings for 8 hours. Add water as necessary.

5. When the puddings are done, remove them from the water. Cool them to room temperature. Remove the towels and foil and re-cover the molds tightly with fresh foil. Store until served.

6. To serve, place mold or molds in a stockpot and pour boiling water to within 4 inches of the top of the mold. Bring to a boil. Cover pot tightly. Reduce heat to lowest point and steam pudding for 2 hours. Add boiling water as needed. Run a knife around the inside of the mold. Place an inverted serving plate firmly over the top, turn them over together as a unit. The pudding should slide out easily.

7. To flambé the pudding, warm ¹/₂ cup of brandy in a small saucepan over low heat. Ignite it with a match, and pour it flaming over the pudding. Plum puddings can be kept up

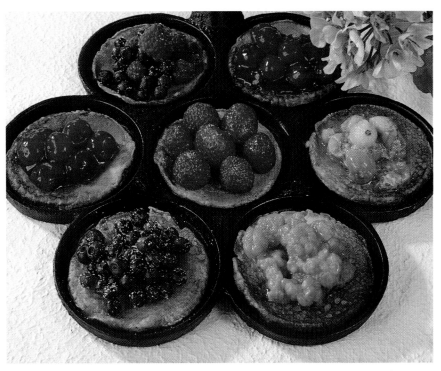

Crepes with Fresh Berries

to a year in the refrigerator or other cool place. Serves 15.

Serving size:	2 ounces
Exchanges:	1 starch/bread
	1 fruit
	1 fat
Calories:	185

CREPES WITH FRESH BERRIES

3 eggs
³/₄ to 1 cup flour
2 cups milk
¹/₂ teaspoon salt
3 tablespoons melted butter
or margarine
Cooking oil
Fresh berries

1. Beat the eggs, flour and a little of the milk together into a smooth batter. Add the rest of the milk, the salt, and melted butter.

2. Pour several drops of oil in a small (5 to 6 inches) frying pan or crepe pan. Heat it so that it almost starts to smoke. Remove pan from the heat and dry it with paper. Pour in the batter so that it just covers the bottom of the pan. Cook the crepes until light brown on both sides.

3. Serve them hot or cold with berries or jam. Serves 40.

NOTE: If making the crepes in advance, store them in aluminum foil.

Serving size:	1 crepe
Exchanges:	1 vegetable
	1 fruit
Calories:	105

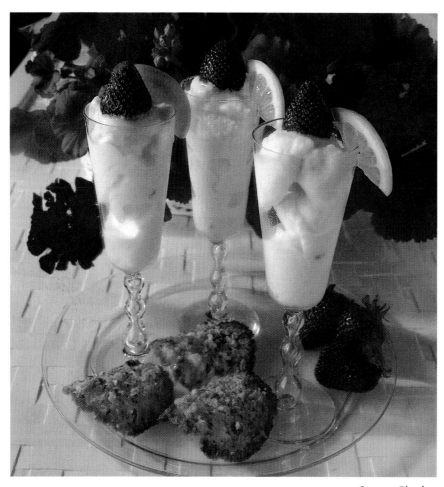

Lemon Sherbet

LEMON SHERBET

3 lemons
3/4 cup confectioners' sugar
1 cup water
2 egg whites
Strawberries for decoration

1. Peel the lemons with a knife. Remove even the white part of the peel. Halve the lemons and remove the seeds. Mix the lemons in a blender or food processor until they become a smooth mass. Add the confectioners' sugar and water. Freeze the sherbet halfway. Beat the mixture several times while it is freezing.

2. Beat the egg whites into dry, stiff peaks. Mix them into half-frozen sherbet. Continue to freeze.

3. When it is time to serve the sherbet, beat it until smooth. Then spoon it into glasses or a bowl. Decorate with strawberries. Serve with small cookies. Serves 4.

Serving size:	4 ounces
Exchanges:	1 starch/bread
	1²/₃ fruit
Calories:	180

CELEBRATION
PUNCHES AND
BEVERAGES

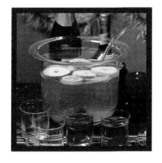

Make a celebration of

holiday beverages. Fill the punch bowl

and serve good cheer in a cup.

EGG NOG

6 large eggs, separated
1 cup sugar
2 cups heavy cream
2 cups 2% milk
1 cup blended whiskey
1/2 cup rum
Nutmeg

1. Place the egg yolks in a large mixing bowl, and beat until pale yellow. Gradually beat in 1/2 cup sugar.

2. Beat the egg whites until stiff, but not dry. Add remaining sugar. Fold the whites into the yolks.

3. Stir in the cream, milk, whiskey, and rum. Mix well. Serve cold with a sprinkling of nutmeg. Serves 8.

Serving size:	4 ounces
Exchanges:	1 1/4 starch/bread
	2 fat
Calories:	190

BLOODY MARY

4 cups tomato juice
1/2 cup beef bouillon
1/2 cup clam juice
Juice of one lemon
Salt and freshly ground black pepper
2 jiggers vodka
1/4 teaspoon celery salt
Hot pepper sauce
Worcestershire sauce
Salt and pepper

1. Combine all ingredients in a tall shaker or pitcher with ice cubes and stir. Serve in tall glasses over ice. Serves 2.

Serving size:	8 ounces
Exchanges:	1/2 starch/bread
Calories:	40

FRUIT JUICE REFRESHER

2 cups grape juice
2 cups apple juice
Large bottle of diet soda water
1/4 cup sugar
Juice of 2 lemons
1 banana sliced
1 cup grapes, peeled and seeded

Egg Nog

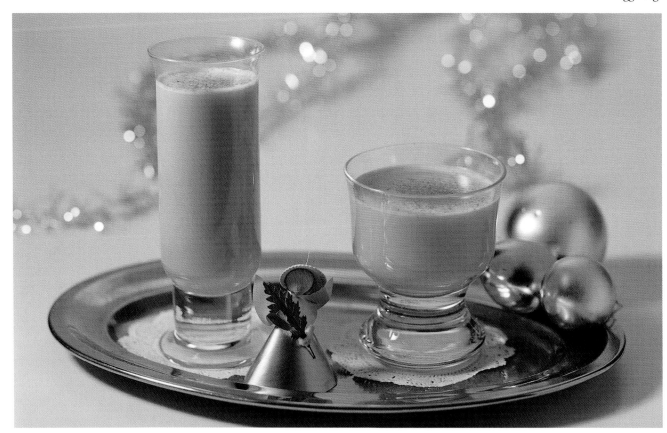

1. Mix the grape juice and apple juice with 2 cups soda water. Set aside to chill thoroughly.

2. Make a syrup with the sugar and 1/2 cup of water. Boil for 5 minutes and let chill.

3. When ready to serve, mix all the ingredients together and top with more soda water. Serves 6.

Serving size:	4 ounces
Exchanges:	1 1/2 fruit
Calories:	90

HOMEMADE APPLE JUICE

5 pounds apples, rinsed and stemmed
1/4 to 1/2 teaspoon ascorbic acid

1. Cut apples into wedges, leaving cores and peels intact. Puree apples in container of food processor or blender. Strain the thick, cloudy juice through cheesecloth. Add ascorbic acid.

2. Pour the juice into suitable freezing containers and freeze. Remember to allow enough time for juice to thaw before serving. Serves 4.

Serving size:	1 cup
Exchanges:	2 fruit
Calories:	120

ICED COFFEE

5 tablespoons instant coffee granules
2 cups hot water
6 cups cold water
Sugar

Vanilla ice milk
Whipped cream
Grated chocolate

1. Dissolve the coffee in the hot water. Add cold water and sugar to taste. Refrigerate until ready to serve.

2. Put a scoop of ice milk into each glass and fill with the iced coffee. Top with cream and a sprinkle of grated chocolate. Serves 8.

Serving size:	4 ounces
Exchanges:	2 starch/bread
	2 fat
Calories:	250

A BROWN, A RED, AND A WHITE

THE BROWN
1/4 pound bitter chocolate
1 cup boiling milk
2 tablespoons sugar
1/3 teaspoon vanilla extract
4 to 5 fresh mint leaves or 1/4 teaspoon mint extract
3/4 cup crushed ice

THE RED
1/4 cup light rum
2 egg whites
1/2 quart fresh berries
2/3 cup water
3/4 cup crushed ice
6 tablespoons sugar

THE WHITE
1 1/4 cups milk
2/3 cup crushed ice
1 tablespoon whiskey or brandy
1/4 teaspoon ground nutmeg

1. To make the brown: Break the chocolate into pieces. Combine chocolate and hot milk in food processor or blender. Add remaining ingredients and puree until the ice has melted. Pour into cold glasses.

2. To make the red: Mix all ingredients in a food processor or mixer. Beat until the ice has melted and the berries are pureed. Pour into cold glasses.

3. To make the white: Pour the milk, ice, and whiskey or brandy into a food processor or blender. Beat until the ice has melted and the milk becomes foamy. Pour into cold glasses, sprinkle with nutmeg, and serve immediately. Serves 6 to 8.

THE BROWN	
Serving size:	3 ounces
Exchanges:	1 vegetable
	2 fruit
	2 fat
Calories:	235

THE RED	
Serving size:	4 ounces
Exchanges:	1 vegetable
	1 fruit
Calories:	85

THE WHITE	
Serving size:	4 ounces
Exchanges:	1 starch/bread
Calories:	80

SPICED MOCHA NIGHTCAP

¹/₄ cup sugar
4 teaspoons instant coffee granules
2 squares (1 ounce each) unsweetened baking chocolate
³/₄ teaspoon ground cinnamon
¹/₄ teaspoon ground nutmeg
¹/₈ teaspoon salt
1 cup water
3 cups milk
Whipped cream

1. Combine sugar, coffee, chocolate, spices, salt, and water in the top of a double boiler over hot water. Stir over low heat until chocolate has melted and the mixture is smooth. Bring to a boil and cook 5 minutes. Stir constantly.

2. Add the milk and heat thoroughly, stirring constantly.

3. When ready to serve, whip until frothy with a beater and pour into serving mugs. Top with whipped cream. Serves 5 to 6.

Serving size:	4 ounces
Exchanges:	1 starch/bread
	1 fat
Calories:	125

HOT CHOCOLATE MEXICAN-STYLE

1-ounce square unsweetened chocolate
¹/₂ teaspoon vanilla extract
1 teaspoon ground cinnamon
¹/₄ cup heavy cream
2 cups milk
2 egg yolks

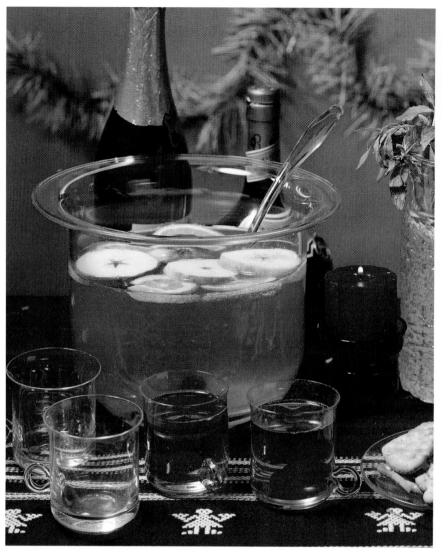

Champagne Punch

2 tablespoons sugar
3 ounces brandy
4 cinnamon sticks

1. Combine chocolate, vanilla, cinnamon, and cream in a medium saucepan. Place over very low heat, stirring until chocolate is melted.

2. Add milk slowly to chocolate mixture, mixing well. Warm over very low heat. Do not allow mixture to boil.

3. Place egg yolks and sugar in a medium mixing bowl and beat until foamy. Slowly pour part of chocolate mixture into egg yolks, beating well.

4. Pour egg yolk mixture back into saucepan, beating constantly to prevent yolks from cooking and setting. Add brandy to chocolate mixture and beat until frothy.

5. Serve hot chocolate immediately in small cups with cinnamon sticks as stirrers. Serves 4.

NOTE: You can make this into an all-family drink by omitting the brandy. Sprinkle with extra cinnamon for a spicier beverage. To make this a richer beverage, substitute 1 cup heavy cream for 1 cup milk. Although this is a dessert drink, you may wish to serve this for a special breakfast or a brunch, or a holiday nightcap.

Serving size:	4 ounces
Exchanges:	1 starch/bread
	1/4 medium-fat meat
	1 fat
Calories:	144

HOT BUTTERED RUM

4 ounces light rum
Juice of 2 small lemons
2 small strips lemon peel
1 cup boiling water
3 teaspoons brown sugar,
firmly packed
1 1/2 tablespoons butter

1. Place long spoons in tall glasses. Pour the rum into the glasses. Add 1/2 of the lemon juice and peel to each glass. Pour enough boiling water into the glass over the handle of the spoon to fill the glass. Stir 1/2 of the brown sugar into each glass. Add the butter; stir until melted.

2. Garnish with a slice of lemon and additional lemon peel, if desired. Serves 2.

Serving size:	1 serving
Exchanges:	1 fruit
	2 fat
Calories:	150

FRUITY WINE PUNCH

2 oranges
1 ripe mango
2 kiwi fruits
1 bottle white wine, chilled
1 1/4 cups dry white vermouth
2 bottles tonic water, chilled
3/4 cup orange juice
Ice cubes

1. Peel one of the oranges, removing as much of the white membrane as possible. Wash the other orange, peel the kiwi, and cut these into thin slices. Peel the mango and cut it into small cubes.

2. Place all the fruit, except the unpeeled orange, in a large bowl or pitcher. Pour in the wine and vermouth. Cover and refrigerate for several hours so fruit absorbs the flavor of the wine.

3. Just before serving, pour in the tonic water and orange juice. Add the sliced unpeeled orange and ice cubes. Serve with a punch spoon in each glass so guests can sample the wine-soaked fruit. Serves 8.

Serving size:	4 ounces
Exchanges:	1 fruit
Calories:	60

CHAMPAGNE PUNCH

Juice of 12 lemons
Confectioners' sugar
1 quart soda water
1 cup maraschino cherries
1 cup orange curacao
1 pint brandy
2 quarts champagne

1. Place lemon juice in a large punch bowl. Add enough sugar to sweeten. Add soda water and ice cubes. Stir well. Then add maraschino cherries, curacao and brandy. Stir well.

2. Just before serving, add the champagne. Stir well. Decorate with fruits in season, and serve in small glasses. Serves 15 to 20.

Serving size:	4 ounces
Exchanges:	1 fruit
Calories:	60

RUM PUNCH

1 bottle light rum
1/2 cup pineapple juice
3/4 cup fresh orange juice
3/4 cup fresh lemon juice
Sugar to taste
3 pints diet ginger ale

1. Combine rum and fruit juices. Add sugar to taste and refrigerate. Add ginger ale just before serving. Serves 8.

Serving size:	4 ounces
Exchanges:	1 vegetable
	1/2 fruit
Calories:	55

HOT APPLE TODDY

8 cups apple juice
1/3 cups brown sugar, firmly packed
1 lemon, thinly sliced
Angostura bitters

1. Combine the apple juice, sugar, and lemon slices in a large saucepan. Bring to a boil. Simmer 5 minutes.

2. Add dash of bitters to taste. Serves 8.

Serving size:	4 ounces
Exchanges:	2 fruit
Calories:	120

MULLED WINE

1/2 cup sugar
1/4 cup water
2 orange slices
6 cloves
2 cinnamon sticks
1/2 cup orange juice
1 bottle red Bordeaux wine

1. Place sugar, water, orange slices, cloves, and cinnamon in a large saucepan. Boil for 5 minutes. Remove from heat. Add the juice and wine. Keep hot but do not boil. Serve with cinnamon sticks or orange slices.

2. Substitute cider for wine, if desired. Sweeten to taste.
Serves 4 to 6.

Serving size:	4 ounces
Exchanges:	1 fruit
Calories:	60

INDEX

A

Almonds
    Alexander Cake, 66
    Squabs Stuffed with Raisins and
        Almonds, 12
Anchovies, Jansson's Temptation, 41
Apple juice
    Apple-Glazed Minted Roast Leg
        of Lamb, 27
    Fruit Juice Refresher, 82–83
    Homemade Apple Juice, 83
    Hot Apple Toddy, 86
Apples
    Apple Crumble, 67
    Apple Pie, 63
    Apple Rice, 71
    Apple Stuffing, 36
    Apple Yummy, 76–77
    Baked Apples with Nutmeg
        Sauce, 76
    Fidget Pie, 47
    Silver Apples, 77
    Sweet Potatoes, Apples, and
        Sausage, 43
Apricots, Roast Duck with Apricot
    Stuffing, 10–11
Asparagus, Marinated Vegetables
    Italiano, 49
Avocado, Stuffed Avocado
    au Gratin, 48

B

Beans, Green Beans a la Grecque, 48
Beef
    Beef Tenderloin Fillets, 16–17
    Roast Beef with Nobis Sauce, 19
    Standing Rib Roast, 17
Beets
    Oven-Roasted Root Vegetables, 44
    Spiced Beets, 47
Berries
    A Brown, a Red, and a White, 83
    Crepes with Fresh Berries, 79

Biscuits, Sweet Cream Biscuits, 33
Breads
    Christmas Tree Bread, 58–59
    Cranberry-Nut Bread, 63
    Dark Date Nut Bread, 62
    Dresden Stollen, 59
    French Buns, 34
    Honey Orange High-Fiber Bread
        Pudding, 67
    Molasses Pumpkin Bread,
        62–63
    New Year's Pretzels, 59
    Pumpkin Bread, 61
    Roasting Pan Bread, 36
    Surprise Pockets, 27
    Tea Bread, 33
    Yankee Spoon Bread, 50
    Yorkshire Pudding, 34
Broccoli
    Broccoli Fritters, 45
    Broccoli-Potato Casserole, 42
    Marinated Vegetables Italiano, 49
Brussels sprouts
    Creamy Brussels Sprouts, 50
    Hot Brussels Sprouts in Dilled
        "Hollandaise" Sauce, 50

C

Cabbage
    Country Cabbage Noodles, 50
    Sauerkraut, 43
    Wild Duck with Red Cabbage, 11
Cake
    Alexander Cake, 66
    Christmas Fruit Loaf, 78
    Christmas Ring, 74–75
    Cinnamon Cake, 68
    Forgotten Meringue Cake, 70
    Fruit Savarin, 74
    Gingerbread, 62
    Old-Fashioned Gingerbread
        Cake, 68
    Orange-Nut Ring, 73

    Plum Pudding, 78–79
    Saffron Advent Cake, 73
    Sand Cake, 68
    Sugar Cake, 66–67
    Yule Log, 70–71
Capon, Roast Capon with Orange
    Pecan Stuffing, 14
Carrots, Oven-Roasted Root
    Vegetables, 44
Casseroles
    Broccoli-Potato Casserole, 42
    Corn Casserole with Ham and
        Cheese, 44
    Eggplant Parmesan, 28
    Epicurean Wild Rice, 42–43
    Fidget Pie, 47
    French Herbed Chicken, 14
    Golden Turnip Pudding, 44–45
    Gratin Vegetables and Noodles, 49
    Holiday Rice, 42
    Jansson's Temptation, 41
    Leeks au Gratin, 38
    Leeks with Mustard Greens and
        Cress, 38–39
    Onion Charlotte, 40–41
    Orange-Baked Chicken, 14
    Oven-Roasted Root Vegetables, 44
    Oysters Baltimore, 32
    Puffed Cauliflower Cheese, 41
    Quick Paella, 24
    Southern Sweet Potato and
        Orange Casserole, 46
    Sweet Potatoes, Apples, and
        Sausage, 43
    Wild Duck with Red Cabbage, 11
    Yankee Spoon Bread, 50
    Yorkshire Pudding, 34
Cauliflower
    Puffed Cauliflower Cheese, 41
    Vegetable Fritters, 46–47
Cheese
    Corn Casserole with Ham and
        Cheese, 44

Eggplant Parmesan, 28
Gratin Vegetables and Noodles, 49
Leeks au Gratin, 38
Pineapple Cheese Pie, 63
Puffed Cauliflower Cheese, 41
Stuffed Avocados au Gratin, 48
Swiss Cheese Soup, 30
Cheesecake, Walnut Cheesecake, 64
Cherries, Cherry-Vanilla Jam, 52
Chestnuts
    Roasted Chestnuts, 44
    Roast Goose with Chestnut-Liver
        Stuffing, 9
Chicken
    French Herbed Chicken, 14
    French Roast Chicken, 15
    Molded Chicken Salad, 16
    Orange-Baked Chicken, 14
Chocolate
    A Brown, a Red, and a White, 83
    Chocolate Meringue Squares, 65
    Chocolate Mousse, 71
    Hot Chocolate Mexican-Style,
        84–85
    Spiced Mocha Nightcap, 84
Clams
    Clam-Stuffed Mushrooms
        Oreganata, 31
    Manhattan Clam Chowder, 30
Coffee
    Coffee Confection, 77
    Iced Coffee, 83
    Spiced Mocha Nightcap, 84
Conserves, Gooseberry Conserve, 54
Cookies
    Christmas Cookie Village, 60
    Corn Flake Kisses, 61
    Gingerbread Christmas Cookies,
        60
Corn
    Corn Bread, Corn, and
        Mushroom Stuffing, 34

Corn Casserole with Ham and
    Cheese, 44
Corn flakes, Corn Flake Kisses, 61
Crabmeat
    Seafood Medley, 23
    Stuffed Pears, 34
Cranberries
    Cranberry Glaze, 8
    Cranberry Holiday Salad, 32–33
    Cranberry-Nut Bread, 63
    Dorothy's Spiced Cranberries,
        54–55
    Pork Roast with Cranberry
        Stuffing, 19
Cream, Sweet Cream Biscuits, 33
Crepes, Crepes with Fresh Berries, 79
Crust, Fresh Game Bird Pie, 12–13
Custard, Custard Pie, 63

D

Dates, Dark Date Nut Bread, 62
Dill, Hot Brussels Sprouts in Dilled
    "Hollandaise" Sauce, 50
Dips, Onion Party Dip, 56
Duck
    Danish Christmas Duck, 10
    Roast Duck with Apricot
        Stuffing, 10–11
    Wild Duck with Red Cabbage, 11

E

Eggplant
    Eggplant Parmesan, 28
    Gratin Vegetables and Noodles, 49
    Vegetable Fritters, 46–47
Eggs
    Egg Nog, 82
    Surprise Pockets, 27

F

Fish
    Fillets of Sole in Mushroom
        Sauce, 24

Flounder Italiano, 23
    Quick Paella, 24
    Seafood Medley, 23
    Smoked Fish Salad, 26

G

Game Bird, Fresh Game Bird Pie,
    12–13
Gingerbread
    Gingerbread, 62
    Gingerbread Christmas Cookies,
        60
    Old-Fashioned Gingerbread
        Cake, 68
Glaze
    Apple-Glazed Minted Roast Leg
        of Lamb, 27
    Cranberry Glaze, 8
    Pineapple-Glazed Baked Ham, 22
Goose, Roast Goose with Chestnut-
    Liver Stuffing, 9
Gooseberries, Gooseberry Conserve,
    54
Grape juice, Fruit Juice Refresher,
    82–83
Gravy
    Roast Goose with Chestnut-Liver
        Stuffing, 9
    Squabs Stuffed with Raisins and
        Almonds, 12
Grouse, Fresh Game Bird Pie, 12–13

H

Ham
    Corn Casserole with Ham and
        Cheese, 44
    Mushrooms Stuffed with Ham,
        30–31
    Pineapple-Glazed Baked Ham, 22
    Rice Salad with Ham, 21
    Southampton Ham, 21
    Stuffed Avocados au Gratin, 48

J

Jam, Cherry-Vanilla Jam, 52

K

Kiwi, Fruity Wine Punch, 85

L

Lamb, Apple-Glazed Minted Roast
   Leg of Lamb, 27
Leeks
   Leeks au Gratin, 38
   Leeks with Mustard Greens and
   Cress, 38–39
Lemon, Lemon Sherbet, 80
Lime, Lime Dessert Fluff, 75

M

Mangoes, Fruity Wine Punch, 85
Marmalade
   Green Tomato Marmalade, 52
   Red Tomato Marmalade, 52
Meringues
   Chocolate Meringue Squares, 65
   Forgotten Meringue Cake, 70
   Spice Meringues, 64
Milk, A Brown, a Red, and a White,
   83
Mincemeat, Rock Cornish Game
   Hens with Mincemeat
   Stuffing, 12
Mixed drinks
   A Brown, a Red, and a White, 83
   Fruit Juice Refresher, 82–83
Mousse, Chocolate Mousse, 71
Mushrooms
   Clam-Stuffed Mushrooms
   Oreganata, 31
   Corn Bread, Corn, and
   Mushroom Stuffing, 34
   Fillets of Sole in Mushroom
   Sauce, 24
   Marinated Mushrooms, 32
   Marinated Vegetables Italiano, 49

Mushrooms Stuffed with Ham,
   30–31
Mustard Greens, Leeks with
   Mustard Greens and Cress,
   38–39

N

Noodles
   Country Cabbage Noodles, 50
   Gratin Vegetables and Noodles, 49

O

Onions
   Onion Charlotte, 40–41
   Onion Party Dip, 56
Oranges
   Crown Roast of Pork with
   Orange Rice, 20
   Fruity Wine Punch, 85
   Honey Orange High-Fiber Bread
   Pudding, 67
   Orange-Baked Chicken, 14
   Orange-Nut Ring, 73
   Roast Capon with Orange Pecan
   Stuffing, 14
   Southern Sweet Potato and
   Orange Casserole, 46
Oysters
   Oysters Baltimore, 32
   Oyster Stuffing, 36–37

P

Parfait, Raspberry Parfait, 75
Parsnips, Oven-Roasted Root
   Vegetables, 44
Partridge, Fresh Game Bird Pie,
   12–13
Pasta
   Country Cabbage Noodles, 50
   Fresh Spinach Pesto, 26
   Gratin Vegetables and Noodles, 49
Pears
   Baked Pears, 72–73

Gingered Pear Ring, 33
   Pear Relish, 52
   Pickled Pears, 54
   Stuffed Pears, 34
Peas, Green Peas with Lettuce, 40
Pecans
   Pecan Pie, 65
   Roanoke Pecan Stuffing, 38
   Roast Capon with Orange Pecan
   Stuffing, 14
Peppers
   Gratin Vegetables and Noodles, 49
   Stuffed Peppers, 23
Pesto, Fresh Spinach Pesto, 26
Pickles
   Pickled Pears, 54
   Spiced Beets, 47
Pie
   Apple Pie, 63
   Custard Pie, 63
   Fidget Pie, 47
   Fresh Game Bird Pie, 12–13
   Pecan Pie, 65
   Pineapple Cheese Pie, 63
Pineapple
   Pineapple Cheese Pie, 63
   Pineapple-Glazed Baked Ham, 22
Pork
   Crown Roast of Pork with
   Orange Rice, 20
   Pork Roast with Cranberry
   Stuffing, 19
   Sausage Meat Stuffing, 37
   Savory Pork in Sweet Potato
   Nests, 20–21
Potatoes
   Broccoli-Potato Casserole, 42
   Fidget Pie, 47
   Jansson's Temptation, 41
   Marinated Vegetables Italiano, 49
Pretzels, New Year's Pretzels, 59
Pumpkin
   Molasses Pumpkin Bread, 62–63

Pumpkin Bread, 61
Punch
  Champagne Punch, 85
  Fruity Wine Punch, 85

R

Raisins, Squabs Stuffed with Raisins
  and Almonds, 12
Raspberry, Raspberry Parfait, 75
Relishes
  Dorothy's Spiced Cranberries,
    54–55
  Pear Relish, 52
  Sonya's Rhubarb Relish, 55
Rhubarb, Sonya's Rhubarb Relish, 55
Rice
  Apple Rice, 71
  Crown Roast of Pork with
    Orange Rice, 20
  Epicurean Wild Rice, 42–43
  Holiday Rice, 42
  Quick Paella, 24
  Rice Salad with Ham, 21
  Wild Rice Stuffing, 38
Rock Cornish Game Hen, Rock
    Cornish Game Hens with
    Mincemeat Stuffing, 12
Rum
  A Brown, a Red, and a White, 83
  Hot Buttered Rum, 85

S

Saffron, Saffron Advent Cake, 73
Salad
  Cranberry Holiday Salad, 32–33
  Gingered Pear Ring, 33
  Leeks with Mustard Greens and
    Cress, 38–39
  Marinated Vegetables Italiano, 49
  Molded Chicken Salad, 16
  Rice Salad with Ham, 21
  Seafood Medley, 23
  Smoked Fish Salad, 26

Stuffed Pears, 34
Salad dressing, French Dressing, 55
Sauce
  Baked Apples with Nutmeg
    Sauce, 76
  Fillets of Sole in Mushroom
    Sauce, 24
  Fresh Spinach Pesto, 26
  Hot Brussels Sprouts in Dilled
    "Hollandaise" Sauce, 50
  Roast Beef with Nobis Sauce, 19
  Stuffed Peppers, 23
Sauerkraut
  Sauerkraut, 43
Sausage, Sweet Potatoes, Apples, and
    Sausage, 43
Sherbet, Lemon Sherbet, 80
Soups
  Manhattan Clam Chowder, 30
  Swiss Cheese Soup, 30
Spinach, Fresh Spinach Pesto, 26
Squab, Squabs Stuffed with Raisins
    and Almonds, 12
Squash
  Gratin Vegetables and Noodles, 49
  Maple Butter Squash, 46
  Spiced Yellow Squash, 48–49
Stuffing
  Apple Stuffing, 36
  Corn Bread, Corn, and
    Mushroom Stuffing, 34
  Danish Christmas Duck, 10
  Oyster Stuffing, 36–37
  Pork Roast with Cranberry
    Stuffing, 19
  Roanoke Pecan Stuffing, 38
  Roast Capon with Orange Pecan
    Stuffing, 14
  Roast Duck with Apricot
    Stuffing, 10–11
  Roast Goose with Chestnut-Liver
    Stuffing, 9
  Roast Turkey with Fruit Stuffing, 8

Rock Cornish Game Hens with
    Mincemeat Stuffing, 12
Sausage Meat Stuffing, 37
Squabs Stuffed with Raisins and
    Almonds, 12
Wild Rice Stuffing, 38
Sweet Potatoes
  Savory Pork in Sweet Potato
    Nests, 20–21
  Southern Sweet Potato and
    Orange Casserole, 46
  Sweet Potato Balls, 43
  Sweet Potatoes, Apples, and
    Sausage, 43

T

Tomatoes
  Gratin Vegetables and Noodles, 49
  Green Tomato Marmalade, 52
  Marinated Vegetables Italiano, 49
  Red Tomato Marmalade, 52
Tomato juice, Bloody Mary, 82
Turkey, Roast Turkey with Fruit
    Stuffing, 8
Turnips, Golden Turnip Pudding,
    44–45

W

Walnuts, Walnut Cheesecake, 64
Wine
  Fruity Wine Punch, 85
  Mulled Wine, 86

Z

Zucchini, Vegetable Fritters, 46–47